OXFORD MEDICAL PUBLICATIONS

Bowel Cancer

THE FACTS

To Peter

with warmest regards.

John

December 1992

Pre-eclampsia: the facts
Chris Redman and Isabel Walker

Rabies: the facts
(second edition) Colin Kaplan,
G. S. Turner and D. A. Warrell

Schizophrenia: the facts
Ming Tsuang

Sexually transmitted diseases:
the facts
David Barlow

Stroke: the facts
F. Clifford Rose and R. Capildeo

Thyroid disease: the facts
(second edition) R. I. S. Bayliss and
W. M. G. Tunbridge

Bowel Cancer

THE FACTS

JOHN M. A. NORTHOVER

Consultant Surgeon, St Mark's Hospital for Diseases of the Rectum and Colon, London, and *Director, Imperial Cancer Research Fund's Colorectal Cancer Unit*

and

JOEL D. KETTNER

Assistant Professor, Departments of Community Health Sciences, Surgery, and Family Medicine, Faculty of Medicine, University of Manitoba, Winnipeg, Manitoba, Canada

OXFORD NEW YORK TOKYO
OXFORD UNIVERSITY PRESS
1992

Oxford University Press, Walton Street, Oxford OX2 6DP
Oxford New York Toronto
Delhi Bombay Calcutta Madras Karachi
Kuala Lumpur Singapore Hong Kong Tokyo
Nairobi Dar es Salaam Cape Town
Melbourne Auckland Madrid
and associated companies in
Berlin Ibadan

Oxford is a trade mark of Oxford University Press

Published in the United States
by Oxford University Press Inc., New York

A catalogue record for this book is available from the British Library

Library of Congress Cataloging in Publication Data
Northover, John.
Bowel cancer : the facts / John M.A. Northover and Joel Kettner.
(Oxford medical publications)
1. Intestines—Cancer—Popular works. I. Kettner, Joel. II. Title.
RC280.I5N67 1992   616.99'4347—dc20   92-12443
ISBN 0-19-261788-5 (hbk.)
ISBN 0-19-262207-2 (pbk.)

Typeset by Downdell, Oxford
Printed and bound in Great Britain
by Biddles Ltd
Guildford and King's Lynn

Preface

WHO IS THIS BOOK FOR?

This book is intended for anyone who would like a broad and up-to-date review of an important disease—bowel cancer. Uppermost in our minds as we wrote this book was the patient him- or herself—as well as close family and friends—who, faced with all the challenges of coping with a serious illness, might be assisted by a familiarity with available knowledge of the disease—its causes, diagnosis, treatment, outlook, and future prospects.

Although written primarily for a 'lay public' without previous knowledge or expertise in the health sciences, we have tried to address some of the broader issues which might be of interest to health professionals who are in a position to present such information to patients (and potential patients) as well as to family and friends of the many thousands of people (for example—25 000 UK citizens and 120 000 Americans) who are diagnosed as having this disease every year.

WHY A BOOK ABOUT BOWEL CANCER?

There are few people who are not aware of lung cancer or breast cancer —but who knows much about cancer of the bowels? More to the point, who *wants* to know?! Bowel cancer? Hardly a conversation topic for teatime, or any other time for that matter. Two taboos in one disease— bowels and cancer.

Perhaps this is why it is one of the least talked about and least-known cancers today—despite the fact that it is one of the 'big three'. It appears that most people do not even know it exists! Even fewer know that it is the number two cancer killer in most Western industrialized countries. Only lung cancer is responsible for more cancer deaths, and it is probably true to say that a non-smoker is more likely to get bowel cancer than lung cancer (since the risk for lung cancer in a non-smoker is only one-tenth that of a smoker). Yet, despite these facts a recent survey in the UK showed that only a small minority of British residents—no more than 10 per cent—included cancer of the bowel (colon) in a list of cancers known to them and, even after prompting, only 43 per cent replied that they were aware of bowel cancer.

It is not the intention of this book, however, to sensationalize nor overstate the importance of bowel cancer nor to give everyone who reads this book a phobia about bowel cancer. The chances are that you will know someone who has suffered from bowel cancer, but will not get it yourself, since less than 5 per cent (one in twenty) of people develop this disease. For most of us, there are more important health problems, such as coronary artery disease, not to mention social and economic problems, which are in more urgent need of resolution. These, of course, are not reasons to ignore bowel cancer—especially if a better understanding of the disease can help us either to avoid it or to improve our chances of surviving and coping with it if we should happen to get it.

A WORD ABOUT THE TITLE

This book is entitled *Bowel cancer: the facts*, which could be misleading and disappointing to any reader expecting to find in it unequivocal knowledge of the cause, diagnosis, and treatment of the disease. *The only certain fact* is that there remain a lot of poorly understood aspects of bowel cancer. Despite a great amount of progress on all fronts, the specific cause(s) are not proven nor are we satisfied with our ability to treat the disease, particularly when it has spread beyond the local area which can be removed safely by the surgeon. We have tried, in this regard, to present fairly 'the facts'—of which there are many—and to discuss openly the current controversies and unknowns.

We very much hope that, by offering a comprehensive and, we trust, easily understandable book on this important subject, those who need to know more will indeed find what they need, and those with no particular personal interest will nevertheless find much of interest in this important and challenging disease.

London   J.M.A.N.
Winnipeg   J.D.K.
1992

Acknowledgements

We must record our gratitude to colleagues and friends who have advised us in those areas in which our own expertise was lacking. Drs Sidney Arnott, Maurice Slevin, and James Foster, and Sister Celia Myers advised on the sections dealing with radiotherapy, chemotherapy, pain relief, and stoma care. Drs Christopher Williams, Clive Bartram and Marie Granowska provided the colonoscopy and scanning pictures. We would also like to thank Mic Rolph for providing the line illustrations. Finally we are very grateful to Oxford University Press for suggesting that we write this book, and to the staff for their patience with our liberal interpretation of production deadlines.

Contents

Plates appear between pages 84 and 85 of the text.

1
The bowel: what it is and what it does

In the later chapters in this book we will look in detail at how bowel cancer develops, what symptoms it may cause, and how it can be treated. In order to understand much of what we will discuss in those sections it is necessary to have a good understanding of the normal anatomy and physiology of the bowel, in other words, what it consists of, where it is situated in the body, and how it works. Only then can we appreciate the effects that cancer, and its treatment, can produce. As we go through this basic description, we will introduce many of the technical terms it will be necessary to know.

According to the *Shorter Oxford English Dictionary* there are as many as five uses of the word 'bowel': *to describe the specific organ*; this use is derived from the Latin word *botellus*, and refers to that part of our anatomy otherwise known as the intestine; *to describe any organ inside the abdomen*, not only the intestines but anything else inside the body, even the womb, a rather imprecise usage as we would see it today, first recorded in 1532; *to describe the most human of all the emotions*, the seat of the tender emotions (pity, feeling, heart) e.g. 'full of guts, and empty of bowels', meaning courageous but inconsiderate; *as a term used by architects and explorers*, the interior of anything ('the bowels of the earth') first coined in 1593; *as a term for our beloved children*, as in Shakespeare's *Measure for Measure*, 'Thine own bowels which do call thee, sire.'

Today we use the word 'bowel' mainly in its medical application to the intestine. The bowel is a very long tube in which the food we eat is digested and absorbed, what is left being returned to the outside world as faeces. The bowel is usually described as consisting of different parts, the so-called 'small' and 'large' bowels. When we talk of bowel cancer, however, we are usually referring to *large* bowel cancer—cancer of the small bowel is a much rarer condition, despite the fact that the 'small' bowel is about four times the length of the large bowel (it is the greater circumference of the large bowel which accounts for its name). This book is solely about cancer of the large bowel. Other terms for the large bowel—more commonly used in the medical world—are the **large intestine**, or the **colon** and **rectum**, its two main subdivisions. The rectum is often considered as the final passageway but that distinction, in fact, belongs to the **anal canal**, the last two inches of the digestive tract, leading to the external opening, the **anus**. The anal canal is not technically part of the rectum and therefore is not usually considered as part of the large bowel. Cancer of the anal canal—even more rare than cancer of the small intestine—is a different cancer yet again and will not be dealt with in this book. However, because of the importance and relevance of the anal canal to the workings of the large bowel, and to the surgical treatment of bowel cancer, it will be described in this chapter.

THE LARGE BOWEL: WHAT IT IS AND WHAT IT DOES

Only about 5–10 per cent of the volume of the solid food we eat finds its way to the large bowel (and eventually out of it!) after passing through the oral cavity (mouth), the pharynx (throat), the oesophagus (gullet), the stomach, and the small bowel. Of these organs, the large bowel, measuring 4–5 feet (about 1½ metres), is second in length only to the small intestine, which is four or five times longer. The main functions of the organs that have handled the food before it gets to the colon are to break it down by both physical and chemical means so that it can be absorbed (particularly by the small bowel) into the blood stream, by which it is taken to all parts of the body to be used as a source of energy, and for growth and structural repair. By the time the remainder reaches the large bowel, most of the nutrients of any value have been absorbed. The undigested contents are no longer sterile (i.e. free of bacteria, as they were in the stomach and upper part of the small bowel) but are now heavily overgrown by the bacteria which normally live in the bowel and which help to digest the food.

The colon, rectum, and anal canal have several tasks to perform. In brief, these are:

- to *absorb* water from the intestinal contents—this decreases the volume to be passed as stool by around 80 per cent;
- to *lubricate* and *propel* the faeces;

- to *store* the faeces until an appropriate time;
- at the appropriate time, to *evacuate* the faeces.

The colon performs the tasks of absorption and propulsion. Storage of the faeces and defaecation are the tasks of the rectum and anal canal, working together. These functions will be described in more detail when the anatomy (structure) of these organs is discussed.

The development of the intestine

It is worth spending a little while thinking about just how the bowel develops in the embryo, because this helps us to understand how it works in the adult.

When the embryo is just a few millimetres long, a straight hollow tube called 'the primitive gut' has already formed. Soon this grows into the beginnings of the series of organs that makes up the adult intestine. As it develops, three areas, called the 'foregut', the 'midgut', and the 'hindgut', can be recognized (Fig. 1), each with its own blood and nerve supplies. We need to know a little about the nerve supply to these parts to understand how we feel pain and other sensations coming from the intestine, producing some of the symptoms of bowel cancer.

The foregut includes the oesophagus (gullet), stomach, and upper part of the small intestine. Trouble in these parts, such as peptic ulcer, may produce a vaguely localized pain high in the abdomen, under the ribs. The midgut, that is, the rest of the small intestine and the first part of the colon, produce a sensation of cramping pain around the umbilicus ('belly button') when these parts are distended with gas, as occurs with the obstruction of the bowel that is sometimes caused by cancer. The hindgut comprises the rest of the colon and rectum. Obstruction due to cancer causes a cramping pain in the lower part of the abdomen.

Each of the three segments of the intestine has its own major artery (each arising from the body's main artery, the aorta) and vein, each of which breaks up into many branches. The foregut has the coeliac (pronounced 'seal-ee-ack') artery, the midgut has the superior mesenteric artery, and the hindgut has the inferior mesenteric artery ('superior' and 'inferior' in this context, by the way, mean 'upper' and 'lower', rather than any reference to quality!). Each artery has corresponding veins, and there are also lymphatic vessels which drain body fluid from the intestine back to the blood stream—these lymphatic vessels are very important also in the spread of cancer. We will discuss these matters in more detail later.

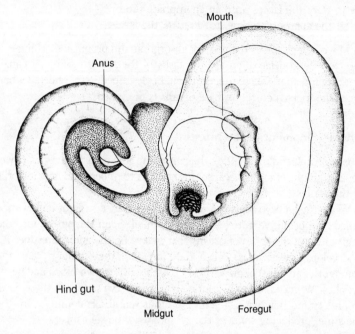

Fig. 1. Human embryo, four weeks after conception. At this stage in its development, when the embryo is little more than one inch long, the intestine from
mouth to anus is already present, and can be divided into the foregut, midgut,
and hindgut. The colon and rectum arise from the lower part of the midgut and
the hindgut.

The abdominal cavity

The intestines and the other organs which play a part in digestion of food
lie in the abdominal cavity, which stretches from as high as the level of
the nipples down to the pelvis (Fig. 2). This cavity is lined by a
membrane called the peritoneum: hence its other name, the peritoneal
cavity. The intestines are packed into this space; some parts can move
around to some extent, while other organs, such as the liver, are held in
position. The peritoneum is a very important part of our anatomy, and
has the following main functions:

● it provides lubrication for the more mobile organs, enabling them to
move and slide over each other with ease;

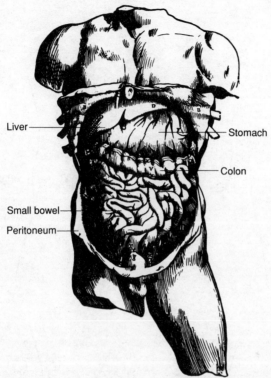

Fig. 2. The abdominal cavity. (Drawn from Vesalius, the Renaissance anatomist). The cavity is lined by a slippery sheet called the peritoneum. The small bowel and, to a lesser extent, the colon and stomach, can move within the abdominal cavity as their muscular outer wall contracts to mix food with digestive juices and to propel the waste products onwards for voiding.

- it contains nerves which are sensitive to inflammation—an important warning when trouble is present;
- it produces fluid containing lymphocytes and antibodies to combat infection;
- in conjunction with the greater omentum (a mobile sheet of fatty tissue which 'hangs' from part of the colon) the peritoneum produces a glue-like material (fibrin) which restricts the spread of infections (peritonitis); (one of the commonest causes of peritonitis is the leakage of contents from the intestines, as can occur when the appendix ruptures during the course of appendicitis or if a cancer causes a leak through the bowel wall).

(a)

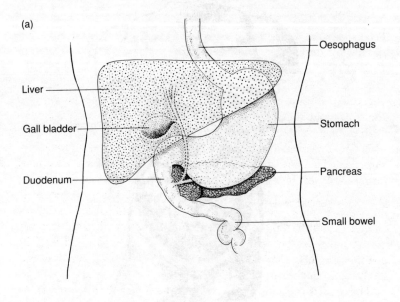

Oesophagus

Liver

Gall bladder

Duodenum

Stomach

Pancreas

Small bowel

(b)

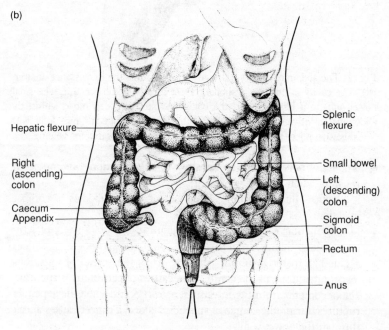

Hepatic flexure

Right
(ascending)
colon

Caecum
Appendix

Splenic
flexure

Small bowel

Left
(descending)
colon

Sigmoid
colon

Rectum

Anus

Digestion and the general arrangement of organs

Food enters the stomach by passing down the oesophagus (which passes downwards through the chest) (Fig. 3a). Here the process of digestion begins; after a short time the partially digested food passes into the duodenum, situated in the centre of the upper abdomen. The liver and pancreas, both situated in the upper abdomen, deliver digestive juices to the duodenum. The food then enters the small bowel, which is around 20 feet long, coiled in the centre of the abdomen, and free to move as it churns the digested food to aid absorption of the nutritious products of digestion. The small bowel is attached to the back of the abdominal cavity by a sheet of tissue called the 'mesentery'. Through this run the arteries, veins, lymphatics and nerves to the bowel. The mesentery, with the small bowel attached along its free edge, has the form of a heavily pleated curtain, as it is short at its attachment to the back of the abdomen (about six inches) but long at its small bowel attachment (20 feet). The lower end of the small bowel opens into the colon in the right, lower part of the abdominal cavity (Fig. 3b).

The colon is generally more fixed in position than the small bowel. At first it passes up the right side of the abdomen ('right, or ascending, colon'), then takes a sharp turn to the left across the upper abdomen ('transverse colon'), and then down the left side ('left, or descending, colon'). After this it forms a mobile loop called the sigmoid colon, then emptying into the rectum, which leaves the abdomen by passing down into the pelvis. Although the colon is mobile to some extent, it is not entirely free to flop around in the abdominal cavity since its right and left portions are fixed fairly firmly to the back wall of the abdominal cavity. In contrast, the transverse colon and sigmoid colon are more mobile, being attached to and receiving their blood supply from sheets of tissue known as mesenteries.

Fig. 3. (*opposite*) Anatomy of the gastrointestinal tract. (a) Upper abdominal digestive organs. Food reaches the stomach via the oesophagus. Acid digestion begins in the stomach, after which the food passes to the duodenum where bile and pancreatic 'juice' are added, prior to entry into the upper small bowel, where digestion is completed and absorption begins. (b) The colon, rectum, and anus. The small bowel empties into the first part of the colon, the caecum. This fluid, containing the 'leftovers' of digestion, is transported through the colon, where most of the water is reabsorbed into the bloodstream. The remainder, i.e. the faeces, are held temporarily in the rectum prior to voiding at a convenient time.

As pointed out earlier, the large bowel is divided into the colon and rectum by anatomists, and these two parts have rather different functions as well. So we will stick with this rather artificial division to describe the large bowel. Let's start with the colon.

What does the colon look like?

For the sake of clearer understanding, the colon is usually described as consisting of the following parts (in the direction of the transit of its contents): caecum ('see-cum'), right (or ascending) colon, hepatic flexure, transverse colon, splenic flexure, left (or descending) colon, and the sigmoid (or pelvic) colon. In reality, of course, it is one single, continuous tube. It is mainly made of soft muscle, about 3–4 millimetres (mm) thick, with a lining of 'mucosa', a special tissue which produces mucus (hence the name) for lubrication, and absorbs water from the bowel contents. The various parts of the colon have special features.

The caecum

This lies in the right lower part of the abdominal cavity; it is the widest and first portion of the colon, and the small bowel empties into it; there is a one-way valve which normally prevents faecal fluid and gas from flowing back into the small intestine. The caecum has the appendix attached to it.

The right colon

The right (or 'ascending') colon runs up the right side of the abdomen to a point under the liver. It is usually bound fairly tightly to the back wall of the abdominal cavity covered on front and sides by peritoneum. The kidney and its *ureter*—the tube draining urine from the kidney to the bladder—lie behind the right colon.

The hepatic flexure

This is the point, lying under the liver, where the colon turns sharply from right to left.

The transverse colon

This part travels across the abdomen from right to left. Lying close to it are many important structures into which tumours of the colon can invade. These include the duodenum (first part of the small intestine), the pancreas and the stomach.

The splenic flexure

The splenic flexure takes an even sharper bend than the hepatic flexure as the transverse colon becomes the left colon. It can be situated quite high under the left ribs; bands of connective tissue hold it to the diaphragm and the spleen (a very blood-rich organ which can be torn easily during surgery on the left colon).

The left colon

The left (descending) colon runs from the splenic flexure down to the sigmoid colon. It lies in front of the left kidney and ureter which must be carefully protected during surgery. When it is necessary to create an artificial opening of the bowel (colostomy) on the front of the abdomen (either temporarily or permanently) it is this part which is most often used.

The sigmoid colon

This is often the longest portion of the colon, named after the Greek letter Σ (sigma) because of the shape of the loop which it forms as it joins the left colon to the rectum at the 'recto–sigmoid junction'. The sigmoid colon is the commonest site for cancer of all the subdivisions of the colon, though rectal cancer is even commoner (Table 1).

Table 1. Distribution of bowel cancer by site

Site of cancer	Percentage of all bowel cancers
Caecum (including appendix)	6
Right colon	3
Hepatic flexure	2
Transverse colon	5
Splenic flexure	3
Left colon	3
Sigmoid colon	21
Rectum	57
Total	100

Some finer points of anatomy of the colon

Blood circulation

After the blood has passed through the lungs to collect a new supply of oxygen, it is pumped by the heart into the body's largest artery, the

aorta, which passes into the abdominal cavity; large branches of this go
to each of the important organs including the bowel, each branch giving
further branches, and so on, ending as the microscopically small blood
vessels, the capillaries. These supply oxygen to all of the abdominal
organs, and absorb digested food and water from the bowel (Fig. 4). The
blood is then collected in veins which join up, ultimately to form the
large 'portal vein', which passes into the liver, where much of the food is
removed and stored. The blood then returns to the heart and lungs to be

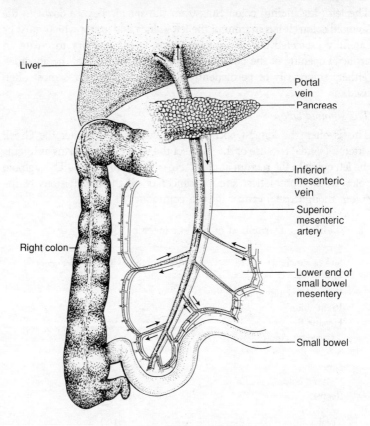

Liver

Portal vein

Pancreas

Inferior mesenteric vein

Superior mesenteric artery

Right colon

Lower end of small bowel mesentery

Small bowel

Fig. 4. Blood supply to the intestines. Blood passes to the small bowel and right
colon via the superior mesenteric artery; after delivering oxygen and collecting
digested food, the blood travels to the liver via the inferior mesenteric vein and
portal vein. The rest of the colon and rectum (not shown here) receive blood via
the inferior mesenteric artery; the inferior mesenteric vein drains into the portal
vein. Cancer cells that have become detached from bowel tumours can reach the
liver by being carried in the bloodstream (the mesenteric and portal veins).

pumped around again. If a cancer has grown in the bowel, cancer cells can gain access to the blood stream in the bowel wall, and can thereby reach the liver, where they can grow into 'secondary' tumours.

Lymph circulation

The lymph circulation is part of the body's defence system, and also serves to collect fluid from all parts of the body (which has leaked from the capillary blood vessels) and return it to the blood circulation. The lymphatic circulation is made up of a massive network of very thin walled tubes which run with the arteries and veins carrying blood to and

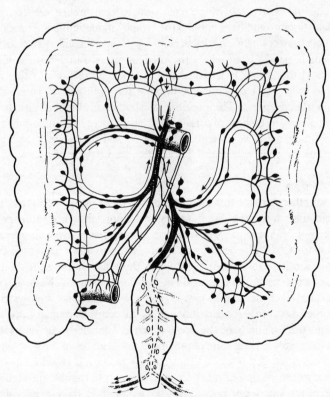

Fig. 5. The lymphatic drainage of the large bowel. Tissue fluid ('lymph') drains from the bowel wall into microscopic lymphatic channels, and onwards to the lymph glands. (The lymph glands are shown as dark spots lying next to the arteries, and the direction of lymph flow is shown by arrows.) Besides ultimately draining lymph back into the bloodstream, the lymphatic channels may carry cancer cells to the lymph glands and onwards to the bloodstream.

from all parts. In cancer patients, the lymphatic vessels may also collect cancer cells from a diseased area, so that cancer can spread in the lymphatic fluid. As in all organs, tiny lymph channels are situated within the wall of the bowel to collect the tissue fluid and deliver it to small glands known as lymph glands which are found very close to the blood vessels supplying the bowel (Fig. 5). There are hundreds of these glands, which have the job of producing 'lymphocytes', cells which fight against germs (bacteria) and other agents which they recognize as 'foreign' to the body. Thus the lymphocytes and other parts of the defence system may be quite important in the body's ability to deal with cancer, by filtering out and destroying cancer cells which have broken off from the primary tumour and have entered the lymph circulation. Sometimes the cancer cells overwhelm the defences and grow into secondary tumours in the lymph glands, from where they can spread onwards into the blood stream as the lymph is returned to the blood circulation. In this way tumour cells can be disseminated to other parts of the body where they may settle and grow. The presence or absence of tumour cells in the lymph glands at the time of surgery for bowel cancer is an important sign to the pathologist, who examines the removed tissue when trying to work out the chances of cure. This is discussed later in the book.

Nerve supply

Like all other parts of the body, the bowel has a nerve supply to carry 'commands' from the brain and spinal cord (the 'central nervous system'—CNS), and to carry messages about what is happening locally back to the CNS. The nerves which carry the sensations from the bowel are not sensitive to the same stimuli as those felt by the skin—touch, heat, or sharpness (as in cutting). The nervous system which supplies the bowel (and all of the internal organs) is the 'autonomic nervous system', so named because its main function is to control automatically and regulate the functions of the body which do not need our direct and conscious involvement. One of the interesting features of the autonomic nervous system is the way it is affected by mood and emotion. Just as anxiety will speed up our heart rate and cause us to tremble through the action of the autonomic nerves, so, too, will it affect the function of the bowel, often in unpredictable ways. Psychological stress may cause diarrhoea or constipation, or be responsible for the production of vague sensations such as 'butterflies in the stomach'. Even chronic pain and other symptoms which seem to arise from the bowel, may be due to psychological and emotional factors for reasons we do not yet understand.

Bowel sensations and pain   The nerves of the bowel are sensitive to the distension caused by a build-up of its contents—particularly flatus (gas or 'wind'). Also, the sensation of discomfort and pain may result from spasms—strong contractions of the muscles of the bowel wall. This can be caused by:

- inflammation of the colon;
- obstruction of the colon, either partial or complete, perhaps due to cancer;
- ischaemia, i.e. reduction or even complete stoppage of the flow of blood to the colon usually because of arteriosclerosis (hardening of the arteries);
- 'functional' bowel disease (irritable bowel syndrome). Functional bowel disease is so named because it appears to be a disturbance of function only; in other words no structural or pathological abnormalities can be found in the bowel. The cause of irritable bowel syndrome is not known, but it is often the only 'diagnosis' which can be made in people with otherwise unexplained bowel symptoms.

Anatomy of the rectum and anal canal

The word 'rectum' is derived from the Latin *rectus*, which means straight. Strictly speaking, however, the rectum is not straight—it has three curves in its total length of about 15 centimetres (cm) (6 inches). It begins at the recto–sigmoid junction and passes downwards through the pelvis to reach the upper end of the anal canal (Fig. 3b). The upper half of the rectum lies in the abdominal cavity while the lower half is in the pelvis. Immediately behind the rectum is the sacrum (the flat bone of the low back, which can be felt between the upper parts of the buttocks) (Fig. 6) and the coccyx ('tailbone'). Sometimes rectal tumours spread backwards to involve the sacrum and the nerves to the pelvis and legs which emerge through it—this can cause very severe pain. The nerves which control the bladder and sexual function also lie close to the rectum.

Some very important structures lie in front of the rectum (Fig. 6). In men, these are from below upwards, the prostate and seminal vesicles (which together produce semen), the vasa deferentia (which carry the sperm from the testicles to the urethra, and are tied off during a vasectomy), the ureters (which carry urine from the kidneys to the bladder), and the urinary bladder itself. In women, the back wall of the vagina lies immediately in front of the lower rectum. The ovaries, Fallopian tubes

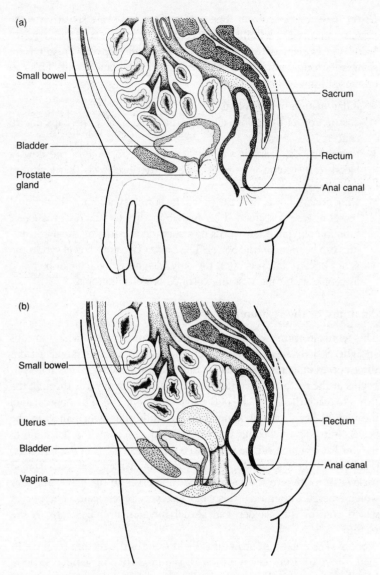

Fig. 6. Important structures in front of the rectum. (a) Male. The small bowel, within the peritoneal cavity, lies in front of the upper rectum. Below the peritoneal cavity the bladder and prostate gland are immediately in front of the rectum. (b) Female. The upper rectum has small bowel in front of it, while the uterus and vagina are in front of the lower half.

and, in both sexes, some of the small bowel lie around the upper part of the rectum, within the abdominal cavity. The close relationship to the rectum of so many important organs poses extra problems for the surgeon in deciding how to tackle some rectal cancers.

Although the anal canal is much shorter than the rectum (about 4 cm —1½ inches) it is a complex structure with important and delicate tasks. It has two developmental origins: its upper half derives from the hindgut and has the same type of epithelial lining, blood supply, lymphatics, and nerves as the rectum. Its lower half is lined by skin, in continuity with the covering of the buttocks. The anal canal is surrounded by the sphincter muscles, whose task it is to maintain continence by constant contraction, while allowing defaecation at the appropriate time by reflex relaxation.

Blood supply, lymphatics, and nerves of the rectum and anal canal

The rectum and anal canal receive their blood mainly from two arteries: the inferior mesenteric and internal iliac arteries. There are other connections between arteries which enable the rectum to receive blood even after surgery has divided these main vessels. Blood returns from the rectum to the circulation, like the rest of the blood from the intestine, via the portal vein to the liver.

The lymph vessels from the rectum travel alongside the blood vessels and proceed in three directions (Fig. 5):

● upwards from the rectum, they accompany the inferior mesenteric vessels and drain into the glands around the aorta;

● laterally (i.e. sideways), they travel to the lymph glands around the internal iliac artery on the side wall of the pelvis;

● downwards, the lower part of the anal canal is drained downwards and forwards into the superficial lymph glands of the groin (where they may be felt by the patient or the doctor) and into the lymph glands around the internal iliac artery. Swollen lymph glands in the groin are caused by many conditions besides cancer; in fact it is quite unusual for bowel cancer to be a cause of enlarged glands in the groin.

The nerve supply of the rectum is similar to that of the colon. It comes from the autonomic nervous system. The rectum is sensitive to pressure and stretching—these nerves make us aware of the status of the rectum —whether it is distended with faeces or flatus, and hence in need of emptying.

Nerve supply of organs around the rectum
The urinary and reproductive organs also receive their nerve supply
from the autonomic system. They tell us when the bladder needs emptying, and control the muscles which achieve this. They also control penile
erection and ejaculation of semen in the male. It is not uncommon for
any or all of these nerves to be severed during surgery for rectal cancer,
as extensive removal of tissues around the rectum may be necessary to
get the best chance of cure. The consequences of surgical interference
with these nerves will be discussed later.

Down the microscope

The appearance of the bowel seen down a microscope reflects its functions. It is organized into two parts: the inner lining ('mucosa') and the
outer wall (muscle tube).

The inner lining of the bowel—the mucosa
The inner lining of the large bowel, known as 'epithelium' or 'mucosa',
contains mucus-producing glands, blood vessels, nerves, lymph
channels, and a thin layer of muscle. The epithelial cells come in contact
with the faecal contents of the bowel, and it is from these cells that bowel
cancer develops. The epithelial cells are fast-growing cells: normally they
have a very short life before they are shed into the faeces within the
passageway of the bowel (the 'lumen') and replaced by new ones. This
feature of rapid growth and turnover may be a factor in the susceptibility
of the bowel to cancer. It is also the reason why the bowel and other parts
of the gut are so sensitive to agents which affect growing and dividing
cells, such as radiation and cancer-killing drugs. Destruction of the epithelial lining of the gut is one of the prominent features of radiation
sickness (from nuclear blasts and accidents), and is one of the reasons for
side-effects from cancer treatments employing drugs or radiation.

The outer layer of the bowel wall—the muscle layer
In fact the bowel has two outer layers of muscle which propel its contents
onwards. It is supplied by 'autonomic' nerves and therefore works
independently of our conscious control. The muscle of the bowel is
relevant to bowel cancer for at least three reasons:

● like all tissues, muscle, itself, can give rise to tumours. Such rare
   tumours, most of which are benign, are known as leiomyomas. The
   even rarer malignant variant is known as a leiomyosarcoma;
● it is important for the pathologist examining a removed bowel cancer

to determine whether the tumour has invaded right through the muscle layer, indicating a worse outlook for the patient;
- the muscle of the rectum and anus is important in bowel emptying: thus, the less of it that is removed at surgery, the better the chance of satisfactory bowel function afterwards.

What does the large bowel do?

As mentioned earlier, the colon serves two main functions: recovery of water from its contents, and propulsion of the resulting faeces to the rectum for timely evacuation.

The colon

Absorption of fluid from the intestinal contents   About one litre (around two pints) of intestinal fluid reaches the colon every day from the small bowel. Of this, normally only about one-fifth is passed as faeces, the remainder is the water absorbed by the colon and returned to the blood stream. A loss of this absorptive ability of the colon (whether due to disease or surgical removal) may result in severe diarrhoea. However, within a week or two of surgical removal of the colon, the lower part of the small bowel usually adapts itself to act like the colon so that the consistency of the bowel motions becomes more normal.

Propulsion of faeces   While absorbing fluid, the colon also propels its contents onwards. This occurs much more slowly in the colon than it does in the small bowel. Although there is wide variation between individuals, it is estimated that fluid will pass through the stomach and small bowel to enter the colon in about four or five hours from the time of swallowing, but it takes two or three times as long to get around the colon. Thus 24 hours is the average time for completion of the journey through the entire digestive tract.

The rectum and anal canal

Despite their important functions, the rectum and anal canal, like the colon, are not vital or essential organs, in other words, we can if necessary live without them. The proof of this is the fact that there are many people who have had them removed, and who are leading normal, happy and productive lives. Nevertheless, natural and problem-free function of the bowels is something which most people take for granted and may not appreciate until they have problems. These problems can be very disruptive and interfere with normal life; fortunately, there have been great advances in our ability to deal with these problems, both in cancer and non-cancer diseases. Following is a brief explanation of the two main functions of the rectum and anus: the storage and expulsion of the faeces and flatus.

Storage of faeces   The main function of the rectum is to store faeces and flatus until the opportunity occurs to empty it. Most people can control the urge to defaecate, and develop an unconscious timetable to fit defaecation into a convenient pattern; others maintain different schedules, while some have no schedule at all.

Expulsion of faeces (defaecation) and flatus   An important task for the rectum and anal canal is to differentiate between flatus and faeces, so that flatus can be passed conveniently and discretely without risking passing faeces unexpectedly. When it is appropriate to pass anything from the rectum, there is a series of events which involves the brain, rectum, anal canal, and the abdominal and pelvic muscles. The process is initiated by a sensation of rectal fullness. Under normal conditions, the urge to pass faeces or flatus is suppressed by conscious activity of the brain until a decision is taken to initiate the process. When faeces are to be passed, it is usual to assume a sitting position (or, in some societies, a squatting position). This straightens out the angle between the rectum and the anal canal, making the emptying of the rectum easier. The abdominal muscles (including the diaphragm) may be voluntarily contracted; as this occurs, the muscles of the anal canal and the pelvic floor automatically relax to allow the passage of faeces, after which they resume their normal state of contraction. The degree of abdominal straining, consistency of the stool, length of the process, degree of regularity, etc., vary greatly between individuals.

SUMMARY

In essence, then, the large bowel is just a long tube made mainly of muscle; it has developed, through anatomical and social evolution, into a very complex organ which can help us to get rid of the body's gaseous and solid wastes as privately and conveniently as possible. We have noted that its lining is the part in which cancer is most likely to develop, that its nerves may give us warnings that disease is developing, and that its blood supply and lymphatic drainage may play a major part in the spread of cancer. Now we should go on to look at what cancer is, and in particular, how it may develop in the bowel.

2
What is 'cancer'?

'Cancer' has become a very common word in our everyday lives; it is a rare family that is not affected in some way by cancer. One-third of people in the Western world will get some form of cancer in their lifetime and it is now the cause of more than one-fifth of all deaths in Western countries. It is unusual for a week to pass without some news in the media about cancer, whether about the latest discovery that something which we enjoy doing or eating causes it, or that a new 'wonder drug' or other treatment is now available. It was often said (until AIDS came along) that cancer was the biggest challenge facing modern medicine. The reasons for this are many, including the fact that cancer has emerged over this century as a disease of increasing importance—now the second leading cause of all deaths (after heart disease). Yet few people would feel confident that they know what cancer is, how best to live their lives to reduce their risk of it (without giving up everything which makes life worth living!), or how to understand and cope with cancer if and when it strikes them, their family or friends.

The word 'cancer' is derived from the *Latin* word for crab and is used in a general way for this disease, whichever organ or part of the body is involved. Carcinoma, a more specific term referring only to those cancers arising from the covering and lining tissues of the body, is derived from *karkinos*, the *Greek* word for crab. Why are these terms derived from ancient words for the crab? There are several possible explanations. The first is that the enlarged veins which may be apparent around a cancerous swelling were thought to resemble the limbs of a crab; another is the appearance of the cut surface of a cancer mass in which the tumour may have the appearance of radiating crab's legs; perhaps a third explanation is the slow leg movements of the crab which conjure up the image of cancer spreading within a person's body.

None of this musing over the origin of the terms helps us, however, to understand what cancer actually is. It is difficult to define simply because there are many types of cancer and because we do not fully understand its causes and its progression once it is present.

(a)

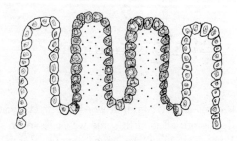

(b)

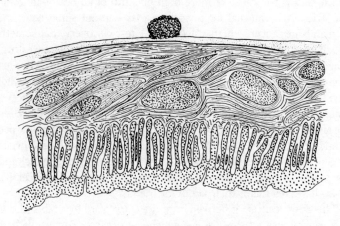

(c)

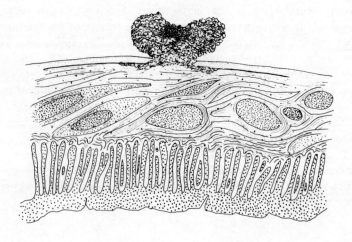

(d)

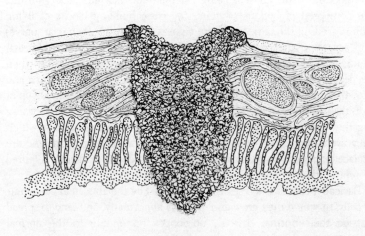

(e)

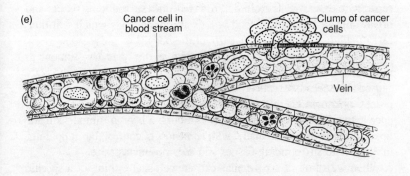

Cancer cell in blood stream

Clump of cancer cells

Vein

Fig. 7. Steps in the development of a bowel cancer. A single bowel-lining cell becomes abnormal and breeds a small clump of similar cells (a). These may grow into a small visible lump (adenoma) (b), which may go on to enlarge into a larger adenoma. This, in turn, may develop an area of true cancer (c), which will then enlarge to destroy the adenoma and begin to spread into the surrounding tissues (d). Cancer cells may enter veins near the tumour and be carried towards the liver (e).

To understand why there are different types of cancer it may be helpful first to consider the actual make up of the human body, our overall architectural plan. Human beings, like all complex animal organisms, are composed of billions of **cells**, the basic building blocks of living things. Cells of the same type form **tissues** (e.g. muscle, bone, fat, nerve) and several tissue types organized together form **organs** (e.g. heart, brain, bowels). Cells grow and divide to form new cells as and when needed under the influence of substances called growth factors and growth inhibitors; so when all is well, tissues and organs are made up of just the right numbers of each type of constituent cell, all working together to perform the complex functions of the tissue or organ of which they are a part. Most cells age, just like the whole organism, and are replaced in an orderly fashion; new cells are produced at the rate required to replace the old ones, this rate varying from tissue to tissue.

Basically, cancer is a disease characterized by the abnormal behaviour of cells, in which they grow and multiply abnormally, and tend to spread outside their normal 'patch', no longer responding to the normal regulatory mechanisms; in other words, a cancer comprises a mass of cells that are growing out of control. Probably starting from a single cell that has become 'malignant', a lump develops which may have the capacity to destroy cells around it, to invade into surrounding tissues and organs and to break into blood vessels and lymphatics which will then carry malignant cells to other parts of the body (Fig. 7).

The cancer at its site of origin is known as the 'primary' tumour to distinguish it from the 'secondary' tumours in other parts of the body caused by spread of cancer cells, usually via the bloodstream—this process is known as 'metastasis'. This helps us to understand the difference between benign and malignant tumours: a benign tumour is made up of cells growing abnormally, with some loss of control, but it does not infiltrate into surrounding tissues and does not metastasize.

When we think of a particular cancer we usually think of a specific organ, e.g. cancer of the skin or cancer of the breast, but it is more correct to think of cancers in terms of the type of tissue from which they arise. For example, the bowel is composed of several types of tissue: epithelium (the inner lining), muscle, nerves, blood vessels, lymph tissue, etc. Although more than 95 per cent of bowel cancers arise from the epithelium, and are therefore classified as carcinomas, there are less common cancers which arise from other tissues of the bowel. Such cancers may behave quite differently and require a different approach to treatment. The classification of cancer is discussed further on p. 25.

Although we classify cancers by the organ and type of tissue in which they develop, it is thought that most cancers arise from changes in a single cell. Such cells multiply until hundreds of thousands of cells constitute a mass which may be noticeable and detectable. For most cancers, this means that the abnormal cells have been growing for several years before they cause symptoms. Sometimes the tumour has meta-stasized to other parts of the body before symptoms due to the primary tumour have been noticed by the patient.

WHAT CAUSES CANCER?

Although many of the parts of the great cancer jigsaw are in place, we don't yet have the whole story. We know that in most cancers the causative factors (whatever they may be) produce changes in one or more of the 100 000 genes which are present in each cell and which control its functions. Certain substances which we take into our bodies, either accidentally or deliberately, may cause very specific damage to particular genes, leading to well-defined functional alterations which in turn lead to 'cells out of control' and hence cancer. In general we do not know the precise modes of action of these damaging substances (collectively known as 'carcinogens') nor are we generally aware of the exact genes that are attacked. A gene which, through the action of a carcinogen, produces a 'malignant' change in cell function is called an 'oncogene'. It has become apparent over the past few years that some gene abnormalities which play a part in cancer development can be inherited from our parents; hence the tendency in some types of cancer for greater numbers to occur in particular 'cancer families'. In most types of cancer it appears that several gene alterations—mostly due to factors taken in from the environment, but some, perhaps inherited—must occur before cell function becomes sufficiently abnormal for a fully blown cancer to develop.

So what cancer-causing agents have we identified? The best known, of course, is tobacco smoke, the 'cause' of about 90 per cent of cases of lung cancer. Yet we do not know exactly how the inhalation of smoke changes normal cells into cancerous cells. Furthermore cigarettes cannot be the whole story in the causation of lung cancer because some people who do not smoke **do** get lung cancer, while most people who do smoke **do not** get lung cancer. In cancer of the cervix it appears that a virus (the human papilloma virus) may be an important causative factor.

The main suspected environmental factors which either cause, or indirectly expose us to the risk of, cancer include life-style factors (certain dietary items, alcohol, tobacco, reproductive and sexual behaviour), occupation, the physical environment (natural radiation and 'unnatural' pollution such as industrial products), infection (certain viruses), and medical procedures (X-rays and other treatments). (See Table 2.)

Table 2. Proportions of all cancer deaths attributed to various factors: from Doll and Peto, *The Causes of Cancer*

Factor	Best estimate (%)	Range of acceptable estimates (%)
Diet	35	10–70
Tobacco	30	25–40
Infection	10	1–?
Reproductive and sexual behaviour	7	1–13
Occupation	4	2–8
Alcohol	3	2–4
Geophysical factors	3	2–4
Pollution	2	<1–5
Medicines and medical procedures	1	0.5–3
Industrial products	<1	<1–2
Unknown	?	?

In 1981 a report to the United States Office of Technology Assessment by two leading British researchers, Doll and Peto, was published by Oxford University Press under the title 'The Causes of Cancer'. In this extensive review of the causes of cancer in the US, it was estimated that the mortality rates due to cancer could be reduced by more than 80 per cent by the removal of known and avoidable causes. These included certain occupations, infections, and polluting agents, but the two most important causes by far were tobacco (30 per cent of all cancer deaths) and diet (35 per cent of all cancer deaths). These estimates were based largely on indirect evidence from the studies of populations (large groups of people with and without cancer). This kind of research is done by cancer epidemiologists (Greek derivation, 'epi' = upon, 'demos' = common people) who try to determine the distribution of cancer—who gets it (old/young, male/female, occupation), where (i.e. geography), and when (cancer rates vary through history). The sort of information which they produce, such as that seen in Table 2, has important consequences for society and how it deals with cancer and health risks. Writers for the general public such as Samuel Epstein of the USA (*The Politics of Cancer*) and Lesley Doyal of the UK (*Cancer in Britain—the Politics of Prevention*), have argued that such estimates, which maximize the importance of life-style factors—smoking, diet, and sex practices (accounting for 80–95 per cent of all cancers)—while minimizing the importance of occupational and environmental factors (5–20 per cent of all cancers), tend to influence opinion towards individual victim-blaming rather than changes in the social and physical environment as solutions to the cancer problem.

To prove rigorously the importance of 'life-style' factors such as the Western diet (high fat, low fibre, low carbohydrate) as a cause in human cancers is very difficult. To identify factors which are responsible for the development of cancer is not the same as understanding how cancer is caused. The epidemiologist may show evidence, for instance, that people who eat a meat-free high-fibre diet are less likely to get bowel cancer, but it is the task of other scientists to determine why and how dietary factors might cause bowel cancer. This requires an understanding of what is happening within the cells, particularly the parts of the cell that control its growth and replication. This is the work of molecular biologists, geneticists, immunologists, microbiologists, biochemists, and many others. Such work will not be further dealt with in general here, although we will return to these topics when we discuss some specific theories of the causes of bowel cancer (see Chapter 3).

TYPES OF CANCER

As mentioned earlier, the body is made up of several different types of tissue. It is useful to classify cancers according to the kind of tissue from which they arise. One reason for this is the fact that cancers which arise from the same types of tissues often behave in similar ways.

The commonest cancers are those which arise from lining and covering tissues (skin, bowel and bladder lining, etc.)—they are collectively called **carcinomas**, although this term is often used interchangeably (and incorrectly!) with cancer. When the lining tissues contain tiny glands which secrete mucus or other substances, the cancer is termed an **adenocarcinoma**. This term covers most tumours arising from the digestive tract, some tumours of the airways, the breast, and the urinary and reproductive systems. Cancers which arise from the supporting structures such as muscle, bone, and connective tissues are classified separately as **sarcomas**. Thus, one type of malignant tumour which arises from bone is called an *osteosarcoma*. Cancers of the blood and immune system are allocated in a separate category: **leukaemia** is the overall term for cancer of the white blood cells and **lymphoma** for cancer of the lymph cells (lymphocytes).

WHAT IS 'BOWEL CANCER'?

Definition

By definition, then, this is simply a cancer which arises from the bowel, or more specifically, in this case, the large bowel. Although there are several tissue types in the bowel—epithelium, muscle, fat, nerves, and blood vessels—the vast majority of bowel cancers originate from the inner lining of the bowel wall, the epithelium or mucosa, which contains the mucus-secreting glands. This part of the bowel wall is in direct contact with the intestinal contents, the faeces, a fact which may be important in the causation of bowel cancer.

Types of bowel cancer

Adenocarcinoma of the large bowel is so much more common than other types or sites of cancer in the bowel that the simpler term 'bowel cancer' or 'colorectal cancer' is taken to mean this particular tumour in everyday medical parlance. Adenocarcinoma of the large bowel may be divided into two subgroups: cancer of the colon and cancer of the rectum, as there are some important differences with respect to diagnosis, treatment, and outcome. To the epidemiologist, concerned with understanding the causes and risk factors for bowel cancer, this division seems to be of much less importance. While there is much speculation about differences in the occurrence and causes of cancer of these two anatomic regions of the large bowel, their similarities are much more apparent. Therefore, for our purposes here, we will regard all bowel cancers as constituting the same disease.

Although more than 90 per cent of bowel cancers arise from glandular tissue, and, therefore, are called adenocarcinomas, there are other types of carcinomas which arise from the lining of the bowel. The significance of these different types is discussed in the section on pathology. There are other much rarer tumours which can arise from the bowel which must be differentiated from carcinomas since their treatment and prognosis may be quite different. These are:

- **Lipoma**—a benign tumour arising from the fat tissue in the bowel. It does not usually grow very large and therefore rarely causes any symptoms, in which case no treatment is required. If troublesome, surgical removal is curative.
- **Leiomyoma**—a benign tumour arising from the muscle of the bowel wall. These tumours do not often cause problems but may bleed causing an alteration in the colour and consistency of the stool. If barium enema (see p. 80) X-rays are used to examine the bowel, it may be difficult to distinguish such tumours from a carcinoma. Surgery is curative since they do not invade tissues or spread from their original site.
- **Leiomyosarcoma**—a rare malignant tumour of the bowel which may be very difficult to distinguish from a carcinoma. It is treated by surgical removal; the patient may benefit from chemotherapy and radiotherapy.
- **Lymphoma**—arising from the lymphatic tissues, this is an uncommon malignant tumour of the large bowel; it is much more common in the small bowel and may arise in multiple sites. Treatment may include surgery but often involves the use of cancer-killing drugs (chemotherapy).

How does bowel cancer begin?

Although the full picture is unclear, it is fairly well established that there are several steps in the transition from normal bowel mucosa to an invasive cancer. It is likely that in the earliest stage a single cell begins to divide to form new cells abnormally, producing a minute cluster with the same high rate of replication. These cells are unlikely to be detectable by any test presently available. After a while the abnormal cells form into a small lump which constitutes a benign tumour known as an 'adenoma' (Fig. 7). Viewed under a microscope, the cells in an adenoma will have certain features which differ from the appearance of normal cells. These differences are referred to as 'dysplasia', which simply means 'abnormal growth'. Most adenomas remain small, never progressing to cause any problem for their host. A few adenomas, however, probably under the influence of further genetic changes in them, induced by other factors, grow into larger adenomas. A proportion of large adenomas take a further step into abnormality when a cluster of cells within them develops into a focus of cancer by invading into the tissues under the superficial layer of mucosa. The cancerous cells then invade locally, destroying what is left of the benign adenoma, and extending down into the muscle layer of the bowel. A truly malignant tumour has now developed (Fig. 7).

This whole train of events is known as the adenoma–carcinoma sequence, and is thought to be the process by which most bowel cancers arise. The evidence that this is so is indirect, but quite compelling. Population-based studies suggest an association between adenomas and bowel cancer, since the rate of occurrence of the two conditions parallel each other. In other words, in areas such as North America and Britain where bowel cancer is relatively common, colorectal adenomas are also common, whereas in Africa or India both conditions are rare. Furthermore, the distribution of adenomas within the bowel is similar to that of cancer, showing a concentration in the sigmoid colon and rectum. Further support for the theory comes from pathological and clinical studies: it is known that larger adenomas are more likely to show abnormal microscopic changes and to contain cancer than small ones. When a pathologist looks closely at a cancer specimen removed at surgery, adenomas are often found to be growing within or beside a cancer, especially the smaller cancers which, presumably, have not had time to grow and destroy the remainder of the adenoma. Furthermore, it appears that people who have adenomas are at a higher risk for developing bowel cancer in the future than people who have not. In one study in which thousands of people had their rectum examined regularly, removing all adenomas, the number of cases of rectal cancer (many years later) was much less than might have been expected; it was speculated (but not proven) that this was due to the removal of adenomas, thus preventing the cancers which would have arisen from them. Further evidence comes from rare cases of individuals with adenomas observed (by X-ray) over many years until they developed into cancers. In the extreme case of the rare inherited condition of familial adenomatous polyposis, in which hundreds or thousands of adenomas carpet the lining of the bowel, it is virtually inevitable that, unless the colon is removed, cancer will develop, (usually before the age of 40), arising, presumably, from one (or often, more) of the adenomas. More recent research involving sophisticated techniques in the laboratory have provided further evidence for this theory by showing abnormalities in the genetic structure of the cells of adenomas which are consistent with cancer-causing potential.

The above observations have led many to believe that adenomas are the precursors of bowel cancer, and this raises the question of whether bowel cancer could be prevented by removing such adenomas before they develop into cancer: a very important and controversial question facing us today. This would be an immense and costly exercise—first of all, adenomas are much more common than bowel cancer (one-third of all people past the age of 60 will be found to have one or more adenomas on thorough examination of their bowel). Our best guess is that less than 5 per cent of all adenomas develop into cancer, and that the time from the origin of an adenoma until the development of cancer averages between five and ten years. So, what should these facts mean in terms of practical policy? As it is technically feasible to find such adenomas and remove them quite safely, should we implement a programme of aggressive detection and removal of adenomas to try to prevent bowel cancer altogether? This question will be discussed in detail later.

How does bowel cancer progress?

It is always difficult to know with much degree of certainty the natural history of a disease, i.e. its pattern of progression once established. To learn this requires the observation of large numbers of patients receiving no treatment or intervention. It is, of course, very difficult for any patient or doctor to agree to this even when it is not clear that the treatments available are providing any benefit. Thus, most of our estimates of the natural course of any disease are crude estimates and usually based on information from a time when no treatment was available. Such information, of course, may not be relevant now since people today are often healthier, better nourished and more able to defend against the threat of disease than they were at the time the natural history was observed.

One natural history study, published in 1964, of the survival of patients with large bowel cancer who did *not* undergo surgical treatment showed how poorly such patients fared. The average survival from time of diagnosis was ten months; less than a quarter of the patients survived more than one year, 10 per cent were alive at two years and only 2 per cent were alive at 5 years. Symptoms had been present for an average of 8.5 months prior to diagnosis. It is difficult to compare the outcomes of such patients (who may not have been typical of all patients at that time) with patients of today who benefit from better family health care, earlier diagnosis, and better treatment. It seems clear, however, that the overall prognosis of today's bowel cancer patient is quite a bit better. At least

30 per cent of such patients (of all ages) are alive five years after
diagnosis, compared to 2 per cent in the old natural history studies in
untreated patients.

Another way in which we witness the natural history of bowel cancer
is to observe how it may have spread prior to treatment, and also the
patterns of spread not amenable to the forms of treatment presently available. The progressing disease manifests itself locally, i.e. at and around
the site of the primary tumour, and as distant spread by metastasis.

Local spread

As the tumour grows, it spreads out through the bowel wall to invade
surrounding organs: the parts at risk will obviously vary depending on
the segment of large bowel harbouring the primary tumour.

In patients with rectal cancer, the other pelvic organs may become
involved. In men, the bladder and prostate are the pelvic organs at risk.
Occasionally a rectal cancer will invade through into the bladder to cause
bleeding or infection in the urine, or even leakage of faeces and flatus into
the bladder (i.e. a 'fistula' has developed) which may be passed in the
urine. In women the vagina and uterus lie between the rectum and
bladder, thus making urinary tract involvement very unusual. Invasion
of the vagina may lead to a fistula, and leakage of faeces from the vagina.
Thankfully these complications are quite uncommon, and are treatable
surgically in most cases. Local spread from rectal cancer may also affect
the small bowel as it lies in the lower abdominal cavity against the front
wall of the rectum, and the side walls of the pelvis where the muscles,
nerves, and bones may be invaded.

Colon cancer may invade the various structures lying behind it on the
back wall of the abdominal cavity, including the ureters and the duodenum. Again, the small bowel, which lies in close contact with the
colon, may be invaded.

Distant spread

The organ most commonly involved in distant spread via the blood
stream is the liver, which will be found to harbour secondary tumours in
around 30 per cent of patients at the time of initial diagnosis; a further
30 per cent are likely to develop liver secondaries at some time after
primary treatment, presumably due to growth from microscopic deposits
of cells already present in the liver at the time of initial diagnosis. Liver
secondaries vary from a single deposit, which may be curable surgically,
to multiple deposits almost completely replacing the liver.

Another important site for spread from bowel cancer is the peritoneal membrane lining the abdominal cavity. Peritoneal deposits develop due to the spread of cells within the abdominal cavity, shed from the surface of the tumour after it has invaded through the full thickness of the bowel wall. Peritoneal deposits may lead to production of a large volume of fluid in the abdominal cavity ('ascites') which may cause marked distension of the abdomen.

The next most common site for distant spread is the lungs, though these are involved in only about 10 per cent of patients, mostly at a very late stage in the disease. If near the surface of the lung, secondary deposits may cause a collection of fluid within the chest cavity, compressing the lung and causing shortness of breath.

Bowel cancer can spread to any other part of the body via the blood stream, though this occurs much less frequently than with the other common primary cancers, arising from the breast and lung.

Pathology—its role in our understanding of the disease and its treatment

Pathology is the branch of medicine concerned with the understanding and description of the process and outcome of disease. Gross pathology is the study of the general appearance of diseased organs or tissues as seen by the naked eye, while histopathology is the study of the abnormal or diseased tissue as seen using a microscope.

The pathologist is involved in the management of the bowel cancer patient at two important stages. The first is to take a close look at any biopsy samples (see Chapter 6, p. 79) from the bowel of the patient to try to establish a diagnosis before a decision about surgery or other treatment is made. The second is to examine and describe the specimen removed at surgery. This involves a naked eye description and a microscopic analysis, which help the surgeon to advise the patient on possible further treatment and on the likelihood of cure.

The pathology can be summarized in a little more detail as follows:

1. **Naked eye description.** This involves a careful investigation of the spread of the tumour, and includes measurements of the cancer, the portion of the bowel and any other tissues or organs removed at surgery. The report may include a photograph and/or drawing of the bowel and the tumour, providing a permanent record for future reference. The specimen is then prepared for further analysis by (1) carefully looking

through the bowel for any other abnormalities such as adenomas or other cancers, (2) taking slices from the primary cancer to examine under the microscope, and (3) finding the lymph glands around the bowel to examine under the microscope.

2. **Microscopic examination.** A detailed description of the following is produced:

(a) The **type of tumour cells**, e.g. adenocarcinoma (the most common by far), signet ring cell (a variant which carries a worse prognosis), or one of other rare types of carcinomas.

(b) The **grade of the tumour** or the degree of 'differentiation' of **the cells** of the tumour. All normal cells of the body are *differentiated* which means that they have developed into the *different* kinds of cells that they are, whether a muscle, nerve, bone, or epithelial (lining) cell. Thus, the degree of differentiation of tumour cells reflects how much the cells resemble the usual appearance of the epithelium (lining tissue) of the bowel. The cells of a **well-differentiated** carcinoma of the bowel resemble the specialized (differentiated) cells of normal epithelial tissue. In contrast the cells of a poorly-differentiated tumour (sometimes called 'anaplastic') do not resemble the normal cells of the epithelium. In general, the outlook ('prognosis') is better for patients whose tumours are better differentiated, i.e. more closely resemble normal tissue, but there are several other factors in prognosis which are of more importance than this.

(c) The **invasion of the tumour** cells and the **body's defence** against it. There are three aspects of importance here, all analogous to the confrontation between the advancing troops of invaders and the resistance of the defenders.

One is the **depth of invasion** into the bowel wall. It has been known for at least fifty years that the outlook is better if the tumour has not broken through the outer surface of the bowel wall.

The second aspect of importance is the nature of the invasive margin of the tumour. More recent research has demonstrated a better outlook for patients whose tumours have a smoother 'expanding' margin than those with tumours whose margins are more 'infiltrating', i.e. projecting through the tissues with finger-like extensions (like a crab's legs—as in cancer, from the Latin for crab).

The third aspect is the mobilization of the body's defence cells, the *lymphocytes*. It has been demonstrated recently that patients with rectal cancers that have a conspicuous presence of lymphocytes at the front lines of the advancing tumour, are more likely to survive their tumour than those who do not. It is not clear whether this is a feature of the tumour or the patient's immune system; in fact, it is likely to be a result of the interaction of the two, and it is this interaction between the 'virulence' of the cancer and the ability of the patient to resist it which is the essence of the struggle (helped, hopefully, by the treatment provided) whose outcome will decide the patient's future.

(d) Another observation of importance is the presence or absence of cancer in the **lymph glands** which surround the bowel and drain the lymph from the lymphatic channels. Patients who do not have cancer cells in the lymph glands (presumably because their defence system has been able to contain the tumour within the bowel) are more likely to do well than those who do have this form of spread. There is some evidence that the number of lymph glands affected is important: recent research in patients with rectal cancer has demonstrated that if the lymph glands contain cancer, it is better to have less than four involved. Presumably, this is an indication of whether the body is in danger of being over-whelmed by the cancer or is still in battle to contain it. This particular feature is the most important in assessing prognosis.

Staging and prognosis

So what does the pathologist do with all this information? Well, first of all, he or she includes it all in the pathology report. Usually, he or she summarizes the information and assigns the patient a classification or 'stage'. This is important for at least three reasons: (1) it helps in the decision-making about whether further treatment (e.g. radiotherapy) is advisable; (2) it improves the precision of the surgeon's attempts to gauge the prognosis (outlook) for the patient; and (3) it aids research into the treatment of bowel cancer by helping to make any comparisons between bowel cancer patients as valid as possible.

The first staging system for bowel cancer was proposed by Cuthbert Dukes of St Mark's Hospital, London, more than fifty years ago. He divided rectal cancers into three stages according to two factors: (1) their depth of invasion into the bowel wall; and (2) the presence or absence of cancer in the lymph glands. His classification is used today for cancers of the colon and rectum and is known as the Dukes staging system (Fig. 8). The stages and the proportions of patients predicted to be alive 5 years

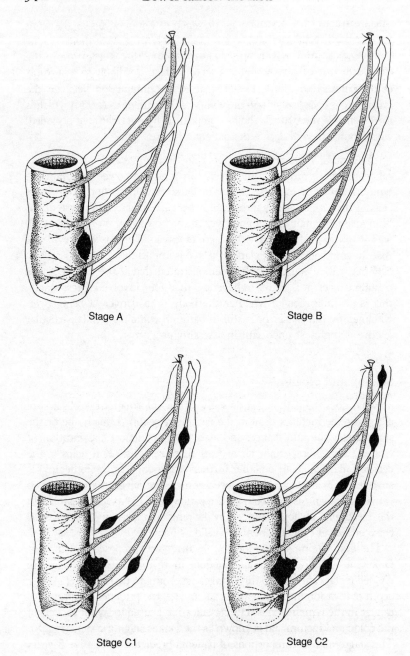

Stage A

Stage B

Stage C1

Stage C2

after treatment (the '5 year survival'), for a group of St Mark's Hospital patients with rectal cancer who had undergone surgery with an attempt to cure (meaning that the surgeon believes he has removed all known and visible cancer), are shown in Table 3. (Five-year survival is taken as the measure of successful outcome because although a few people may develop recurrence after that stage, for most the risk has diminished almost to zero.)

Table 3. Predicted percentage of patients who will survive for 5 years (rectal cancer patients at St Mark's Hospital)

Dukes' stage	Bowel wall invasion	Lymph gland status	5-year survival
Stage A	Contained within	No cancer	97%
Stage B	Through bowel wall	No cancer	81%
Stage C1	Any degree of local spread	Cancer present, but not in the highest gland	51%
Stage C2	Any degree of local spread	Cancer in highest (apical) gland	23%

The figures in this table show the usefulness of these factors for predicting the probability of survival. Even for the worst category (C2), one in four patients will survive. It is important to keep in mind that the figures in the table are for a very select group of patients, and are not applicable to all people with bowel cancer. First, these are patients with rectal cancer: the prognosis for patients with cancer of the colon is not

---

Fig. 8. (*opposite*) Dukes' pathological staging system. This is a scheme whereby a pathologist can predict the possible future of the patient after surgery for bowel cancer. **Stage A.** Primary cancer has not spread through the bowel wall muscle layer, and no lymph glands are involved. This stage carries a very good outlook ('prognosis'). **Stage B.** The primary cancer extends right through the bowel wall, but no lymph glands are involved. **Stage C.** Whatever the extent of the primary tumour, if any of the lymph glands are involved, the tumour is at stage C. If the lymph gland furthest away from the primary tumour contains cancer, this is stage C2, and signifies a very poor outlook. Lesser degrees of lymph gland involvement constitute stage C1, which carries a slightly better prognosis.

exactly the same. Second, these are patients who have undergone treatment aimed at cure, i.e., they have no evidence of spread of disease beyond the limits of surgical clearance at the time of operation. Thirdly, they were all selected for treatment at a specialty hospital for diseases of the bowel. Partly because of the selection process through which information is published, such results are usually more favourable and optimistic than the whole picture based on the routine collection of national (or other population-based) statistics. For all these reasons, it is important to look at national statistics rather than the experience of one group of patients or one hospital if one wants to get a more representative picture of the situation. Such information is available from the cancer registration statistics of the Office of Population Censuses and Surveys of England and Wales as well as many other countries which collect such data. Although there has been a trend of improvement in 5-year survival over the years, the overall 5-year *relative* survival (which takes account of deaths expected from other causes) of patients diagnosed in the 1970s was 30 per cent, that is, less than one-third of all patients with bowel cancer diagnosed at that time were alive 5 years later.

SUMMARY

We have seen that cancer is basically a disease of abnormal cell growth and control. We know some of the mechanisms by which it may arise, and we can recognize aspects of the behaviour of individual cancers which help us to forecast the outcome of the disease in individual patients.

Next we must look in more detail at what is known of the mechanisms of development of bowel cancer (carcinogenesis).

3
The causes of bowel cancer

Although improvements in the treatment of a disease should decrease the pain and suffering caused by it, prevention would of course be far better. In order to prevent a disease, we have to develop a good understanding of its causes so that we can take the necessary counteraction. So what are the causes of bowel cancer, and how might we use this knowledge in prevention?

The short answer to this question is that, on the data presently available, we don't know for sure—to use the legal analogy, the evidence to hand might get the case to court, but no jury would be persuaded that the case was proven 'beyond reasonable doubt'. Nevertheless, large volumes of evidence are available, and deserve careful review.

It has been estimated that a quarter of a million people around the world die every year from bowel cancer. This is despite the fact that the disease is rare amongst the majority of the world's people who live in Africa, Asia, and much of South America. The disease is commonest in western Europe, North America, Australasia, South Africa, and the countries around the River Plate in South America. In the UK, for instance, with a population of 55 million, there are about 17 000 deaths and 25 000 new cases of bowel cancer per year; it accounts for about 10 per cent of all cancer deaths and is second only to cancer of the lung. In comparison to all causes of death, bowel cancer is the primary cause for 3 per cent of the British population. Thus, although it is one of the ten leading specific causes of death in most industrialized societies, it ranks well behind diseases of the circulation—mainly coronary heart disease (heart attacks) and cerebrovascular accidents (strokes) which are responsible for more than 10 times the number of deaths. About 1 in 25 British residents will get bowel cancer in their lifetime. Within areas of relatively high incidence there are variations: it is commoner in Scotland and Ireland than the rest of the British Isles, and in the northern parts of the US compared to the South. A quick look at the graph below which shows lifetime risk ('cumulative incidence') of developing bowel cancer will give some idea of the range of risk around the world. Residents of Bombay, for instance, have one-seventh of the risk for this disease compared to people living in the north-eastern United States. All this indicates that, by and large, bowel cancer is a disease of the 'Western', 'developed', industrialized regions.

Cumulative Incidence of Colorectal Cancer in 15 Countries

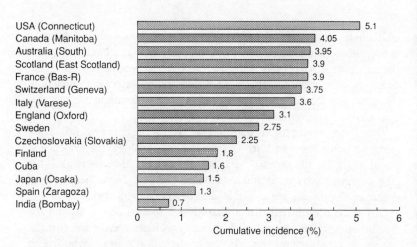

What does this tell us about the causes of the disease? Is there something different about the high and low risk people, or about where they live? Might it mean that the high risk peoples of the industrialized countries have something wrong in their genetic make-up? A parallel for this is the high risk of sickle cell anaemia in Blacks compared to other races: this disease is exclusively due to a genetic abnormality. But there is good evidence that the main causes of bowel cancer are *not* inborn. We need look no further than those people who have 'migrated' from low risk areas to high risk countries—the Black slaves and their descendants who now live in the US, and the Japanese who moved to Hawaii and the US West Coast are good examples. These people took on the risk level of their adopted countries, strongly suggesting that it was their new environment rather than themselves that generated the risk for this disease. If more evidence is wanted, we should note the increasing incidence of the disease in countries, or parts of countries, which are 'westernizing'.

If the causes of bowel cancer are mainly related to something other than genetic make-up, we can describe them as being 'environmental', that is, the causes are likely to be found in circumstances, habits, and life-style. But this covers a multitude of possibilities. First we could look at environmental factors in two groups, those which the whole population shares, and those which vary between economic, cultural, religious, and other groups within a country. And here we find another important clue— bowel cancer is more common in the richer, urbanized members of the population of 'low risk' countries. So it is unlikely that shared factors such as sunlight, climate, air pollution, etc., are important as these would have a more equal effect across the populace. So what about the 'individual environment'? What about personal circumstances, hygiene, sexual activity, etc? What about smoking and other addictive agents? All of these factors have been implicated in some form of cancer. Cervical and anal cancer seem related to sexual activity, mouth and gullet cancer are caused in vast numbers by chewing the betel nut in India and other Asian countries. And we all know about smoking and lung cancer. But there is no evidence that any of these factors is important in the causation of bowel cancer. So what environmental factors are we left with? The short answer is our diet, and a slightly longer answer is what we eat and how we digest it. After all, the bowel lining, where cancer develops, has the substances which digest our food (and this includes the myriad of bacteria which live in the bowel and which aid the digestive process), and the products of digestion, as its most intimate environmental neighbours. For many years now, the highly refined diet born of industrialized agriculture and food processing has been the number one suspect in the hunt for the causes of bowel cancer.

If the 'Western' refined diet is culpable, it could be expected that the disease became more prevalent in 'Western' countries as this diet evolved: in other words, is bowel cancer a new disease? Are any items of diet particularly related to cancer risk? And if possible, we need to work out precisely how any highly suspect food items might produce a cancer.

IS BOWEL CANCER A 'NEW' DISEASE?

Is bowel cancer a new disease which has come about because of new causative factors in the environment, or has it been with humans for all time? This is a difficult question to answer. It is difficult to observe trends over long periods of time since most countries have not long kept records of the number of people who get or die from bowel cancer. Those who believe that it is a disease caused by the modern Western high-fat, low-fibre diet argue that the low incidence of the disease in countries where the diet still resembles that of the earlier prehistoric hunter-gatherer societies suggests that it is a disease that used to be less common than it is today. In 1987, Cohen published an article in *Scientific American* in which he tried to compare the average Western diet today with that of our prehistoric 'hunter-gatherer' ancestors. Table 4 summarizes his findings.

Table 4. Comparison of average contemporary Western diet with that of 'hunter-gatherer' ancestors

Food type	Then (hunter-gatherers)	Now (Western)
Fat (% of calories)	20%	40%
Unsaturated/saturated fats	Higher	Lower
Fibre intake	45 g/day	15 g/day
Ascorbic acid, calcium	Higher	Lower
Complex carbohydrates	Higher	Lower
Refined sugars	Lower	Higher

It seems fairly certain that the essential items in the diet of our ancestors remained unchanged for thousands of years, only to be revolutionized as cities developed in response to industrialization. Where this occurred earliest, and of course Britain leads in this league table, the dietary changes are the most established. In most countries where records are available, it is interesting to note that the incidence (that is the rate of new cases) has changed little over 70 years. If there is any trend in countries like the UK and the US, it is a slight trend of increasing incidence. A comparison of trends of bowel cancer mortality over time reveals another interesting pattern—countries whose rates were low 20 or 30 years ago (e.g. Japan, Yugoslavia) are rising by as much as 5 per cent per year, in parallel with their development as industrialized nations.

If bowel cancer has grown in incidence as industrialization has become established, are any of the dietary differences shown in the table above, acting singly or together, responsible factors in the causation of bowel cancer?

IS IT WHAT WE EAT?

Several dietary items have been under suspicion for a long time, and the evidence has been accumulating slowly. It is important to emphasize at this point that the evidence is largely circumstantial, so that it is impossible to give firm dietary advice which we *know* would decrease the risk of bowel cancer. We have yet to reach a stage comparable with the widely accepted culpability of smoking in lung cancer. There are several types of scientific study which have been performed to hunt for evidence of dietary causes of bowel cancer:

1. **Population studies.** In these, diet is compared between whole populations; we have already heard a little about data from such studies. The problem with this approach is that the evidence is rather 'soft': trying to record and describe the diet for large numbers of people is difficult, while the cancer incidence data may be inaccurate from some countries, especially those with little to spend on luxuries like cancer statistics.

2. **Case-control studies.** These involve identifying individuals with bowel cancer (the 'cases'), finding others who *do not* have bowel cancer but are otherwise much like the cases in terms of age, income, occupation, residence, etc. (the 'controls'), and comparing their diets. A major problem here is that the presence of cancer in the cases may change their appetite and preferences, so that their prevailing diet may differ markedly from the one they were taking while the cancer was developing (clearly the more important diet).

3. **Cohort studies.** In the Roman army, a 'cohort' was a small body of soldiers. In medical research parlance, a 'cohort' is a relatively small group of people who, for instance, may be suffering from an ill-understood disease, and who are being closely watched to check on the progress of the disease, in order to learn more about it. Or they may, as in this case, be a group of apparently healthy individuals whose diets are recorded, after which their health is monitored for a long period, say ten years. At the end of this time the diet of any that have developed bowel cancer is compared with those who have not. This is perhaps the most accurate and informative method of checking possible relationships between diet and bowel cancer, but it is very time-consuming and expensive.

Having said all this, there are consistent strands which have emerged from many studies performed over the years. It's worth looking at, and testing the strength of, the evidence suggesting a role for:

● low dietary fibre
● high dietary fat

as possible factors in the causation of bowel cancer.

Low dietary fibre

Dietary fibre is a broadly-used term for substances of plant origin which are *not* metabolized (changed and/or broken down), by the enzymes and other digestive secretions of the intestine. Our usual sources include the bran of wheat (from the husk of the seed) and the fibrous parts of fruit and vegetables. Since they are not metabolized, they make up a large part of the undigested substance of the stool which is finally excreted as waste. On first impression it would seem unlikely that a food substance which is not metabolized or absorbed into our bodies to be used for energy expenditure or body-building and growth, and is merely excreted, could be important to our health! Yet many believe that increasing the fibre content of our diet is one of the single most important preventive measures we can take: not only against bowel cancer but many other diseases as well. Over many decades there have been medical writers, including Arbuthnot-Lane and Allinson (of bread fame), who have extolled the virtues of the fibre content of the diet as a health-giving measure. In 1971, Denis Burkitt, an English surgeon who worked in Africa, published a classic paper on the epidemiology of cancer of the colon and rectum. Based on his own studies and observations, as well as those of others, Burkitt concluded that diet was the main cause of bowel cancer (and several other conditions of the bowel such as piles and diverticular disease, as well as other diseases like diabetes and varicose veins). He hypothesized that the adoption in the Western world of a diet high in refined carbohydrate but low in unrefined fibre, was the most important responsible factor and warned against the danger of removing so much unabsorbable fibre from our food and the associated over-ingestion of refined carbohydrates.

Ideas such as these are still the basis of many present-day theories and controversies. However the 'fibre is good for you' hypothesis has not been proven and remains controversial.

Besides drawing on the thoughts of those who went before him, how did Burkitt arrive at his conclusions? He was struck by the fact that so few of his African patients suffered from the diseases so common in the UK and the Western world, including bowel cancer. Observing that

American Blacks were as likely to get bowel cancer as American Whites, he concluded that the differences must be environmental rather than genetic. Assuming that conditions within the lumen of the bowel would affect the environment of the mucosa (lining) of the bowel more than substances reaching the bowel from the bloodstream, he focused his attention on features of the diet and the faeces which might explain the differences in disease occurrence. He observed several differences between the faeces and bowel function of Africans and Westerners which he attributed to differences in the diet.

His observations confirmed what others had recorded:

- The stools of those eating high fibre diets are almost invariably bulky, soft, and non-odorous in comparison to the formed and often faceted motions so common in communities eating highly processed food.

- The relative absence of fetid smell in the stools of people in developing communities and in the stools of wild animals, is also significant and is believed to indicate a lower rate of bacterial decomposition compared to that occurring in Western countries.

- By having people swallow special plastic pellets which can be detected by X-ray or by washing the stool through a wire mesh, the transit time (time it takes for substances to make their way through the digestive tract and out) could be measured and compared. He found that it took English boarding school boys more than twice as long as African villagers to pass the markers. He also weighed the stools of subjects on different diets and observed that the average daily weight of stool of African villagers was 450 grams—more than three times that of boys at an English boarding school. In another comparison of Africans living on different diets using ingested dyes, he noted that it took twice as long for the dye to be passed by African medical students on a refined diet as it did for African miners on traditional African diet. Half-way in between were African trainee-teachers on a mixed diet.

- The fact that bowel cancer and other diseases of the bowel have their greatest incidence in the segment of bowel in which faecal propulsion is slowest, contact time with the bowel is longest, and bacterial counts are highest (the sigmoid colon and the rectum), suggests a relationship between these diseases and bowel content.

- The altered bacterial content of stools may lead to cancer-promoting degradation of bile salts (which are produced in the liver and excreted into the digestive tract via the gall bladder and the bile ducts). Burkitt noted that the breakdown products of bile acids had already been shown to be cancer-promoters. Noting observations that the quantity of bile acids is greater in the stools of Africans on a high fibre diet than in Europeans on diets with reduced fibre content, Burkitt argued that this was because of abnormal or excessive bacterial growth in the intestine (due to the Western diet) converting the bile acids into carcinogenic (cancer-causing) by-products.

- The effects of any cancer-causing agents in the faeces would be maximized by anything which might prolong contact with the mucosa, namely concentration in the faeces and length of time in contact. The higher concentration of stool content and the slower transit associated with the low-fibre diet, would both increase this contact.

Burkitt's publications, though not original in their concepts, nevertheless captured the attention of doctors and others interested in preventive medicine, and made quite an impact on the debate about the causes of colorectal cancer (and many other conditions). Since his work, there have been many other studies (using all the methods discussed earlier) which support the concept of low dietary fibre as a predisposing factor to bowel cancer. Supporters of the fibre theory have had a great impact on the life-style of many people who have joined the 'muesli-generation'. Yet the evidence for a direct relationship between fibre intake and bowel cancer remains largely circumstantial; major reviews of the evidence have come to very different conclusions. For instance, in 1982 the Committee of the National Academy of Sciences of the USA was sceptical, reporting that, 'The committee found no conclusive evidence that dietary fibre (such as that present in fruits, vegetables, grains, and cereals) exerts a protective effect against colorectal cancer in humans'. In 1987, however, after an exhaustive and critical review of the medical literature, researchers at the US National Cancer Institute considered that the vast amount of data from several different sorts of scientific study offered support for the fibre theory. Their key conclusions were:

- 'Dietary fibre and its interaction with fat remains the single most comprehensive explanation of the causation of bowel cancer', but that:
- 'The causal mechanisms of bowel cancer clearly involve more than low-fibre diets.'

The debate has been helpful for those who produce and distribute fibre-rich foods, but its value for the ingesters of bran and the like has yet to be proven fully. For the moment, if you are someone who opts for things which may make you more healthy or may protect you, you will be one of the millions who go for high-fibre foods.

High dietary fat

Countries which have a high incidence of bowel cancer also consume large amounts of meat and animal fat. This is not sufficient evidence for a cause and effect explanation, since there are other factors common to these countries which may be responsible. Several case-control and cohort studies have examined this question, and have shown a relationship between total fat consumption and bowel cancer risk. It seems likely that the effect of fat is not direct (fat itself does not cause cancers to appear or grow) but indirect, by its stimulation of the liver to produce bile acids and cholesterol.

What are 'bile acids', and what is their role in bowel cancer?
We said earlier that the environment of the bowel lining included the substances which help to digest our food and the bacteria that live in the bowel normally, and which also help in the digestive process. It seems highly likely that substances called bile acids may play a part in the development of bowel cancer.

Bile acids and cholesterol are produced in the liver, and passed into the intestine in bile. Bile acids play an important part in fat digestion by breaking it up into minute globules ('emulsification') which are easier to digest and absorb; in fact, the presence of fat in the intestine encourages the liver to produce more bile acids to promote its digestion. The more fat that is eaten, the more bile acids are sent into the bowel to deal with the load. It appears that certain bacteria in the bowel are able to convert the bile acids and cholesterol from the form produced by the liver into a different form which then can actively promote the growth of existing small adenomas into larger ones, which are more likely to develop into cancers. It is very likely that these cancer-promoting substances produced in the bowel have a direct effect on the bowel lining cells, as the contents of the colon and rectum lie in contact with the lining. It is also likely that the longer the contact goes on, the greater the cancer-promoting effect. So those parts of the bowel which store faeces for the longest periods are the areas most likely to develop large adenomas and cancers. This is the theory behind the fact that more cancers develop in the sigmoid colon and rectum, those areas which spend most time in direct contact with faeces and hence with the bile acids.

Cancer promoters and cancer initiators

In that last section we used the term 'cancer promoter' to describe the
substances produced in the bowel which encourage the growth of small
adenomas into larger ones, and hence into cancers. You might well ask
what causes the *first* step, the development of the small adenoma from
normal bowel mucosa? These substances could be called 'cancer initi-
ators'; it is likely that they comprise a variety of substances which are
widely present in very low concentration in our environment, including
food. Acting over many years these substances probably start the train of
events which, in those eating a 'Western' diet, lays the ground for the
events described above.

Can anything else in our diet affect the development of bowel cancer?

Vegetables

Of course, people who eat less meat tend to eat more vegetables, and it is
possible that any reduction in risk for bowel cancer among non-meat
eaters is due to a protective effect of vegetables, and this may be due to
more than their fibre content. Some animal research has shown that
addition of cruciferous vegetables (broccoli, brussel sprouts, cauliflower,
etc.) can protect against certain cancers. Some case–control studies in
humans have also shown that the risk of bowel cancer can be reduced by
as much as 25 per cent in people who eat large amounts of vegetables.
Some of the vegetable effect is likely to be due to the fibre found in many
types, but a 'chemoprotective' effect may occur due to the presence of
certain other substances (see next section).

Vitamins and trace elements

There is evidence that certain vitamins and so-called 'trace elements'—
substances present in the body in minute amounts which play a crucial
part in the workings of the body—may help to prevent, or slow the
growth of, tumours. Vitamin A (retinol), Vitamin C, calcium, and
selenium have all been mentioned in this context. At present, the data
suggesting 'chemopreventive' roles for these substances have come
mainly from studies of tumours in animals, though there are studies
under way to look at their role in humans, particularly in the prevention
or inhibition of growth of adenomas in those who have already been
treated for this problem. We will have to await the results of these studies
before anything further can be said.

Summary—diet and bowel cancer

There are lots of unanswered questions in this complex scientific story. But the most likely series of events leading to bowel cancer includes the initiation of small adenomas by environmental carcinogens, and the growth of some of these in the appropriate conditions to form large adenomas, and then cancer. These stages are encouraged by dietary fat, which increases the amount of bile acids and cholesterol in the bowel. These substances are acted upon by bacteria to produce cancer promoters. Some food constituents, particularly fibre, mollify the effects of the promoters, in the case of fibre by hurrying them out of the bowel.

GENES AND BOWEL CANCER

So much for the environmental agents which are thought to play the largest part in the development of bowel cancer. We have known for a long time that diet and the environment are not the whole story: in particular, we have known for decades that our genetic make-up may predispose us to bowel cancer. Of late, this has become a very important area of research, and has given us insight into the way in which environmental agents might actually achieve their effects.

Our earliest inkling that increased risk of bowel cancer could be passed downwards within families came with the recognition of the rare condition of **familial adenomatous polyposis**. Those who inherit this disease (and half the offspring of an affected person are likely to inherit it) carry a 100 per cent risk for bowel cancer if not treated to try to prevent malignancy (see p. 84). Other more common patterns of family occurrence suggest that genetic factors may play a role in up to 25 per cent of all cases of bowel cancer, but this is very difficult to prove, partly because the mere occurrence of bowel cancer within families does not necessarily imply that the cause is genetic. Families tend to experience the same environment (diet, culture, life-style, etc.), and any patterns of disease which may be found may be more the result of a shared environment than shared genes: one way in which this difficult problem can be investigated is to look at the spouses (as well as blood relatives) of cases of the disease, who presumably share any environmental risks. If children or parents seem to share a risk while spouses do not, this is taken as evidence of genetic rather than environmental causative factors.

To understand this issue better, we must be clear about what is meant by 'genetic cause' of a disease. We know that the genes are the 'engineering plans' of the cell, the molecular code which instructs our cells to give rise to human parts and processes, as opposed to those which would be of more use to a giraffe or a sunflower! What, then, does it mean to say that we are born with genes which instruct our cells to become cancerous? And, if this were the case, why would such genes be passed on from generation to generation?

The answer to the latter question is fairly easy—any disease which does not interfere with the ability to have children and pass on our genes to the next generation will do just that—be passed on. Even if bowel cancer were a uniformly fatal disease (which it certainly isn't), by the time the disease develops, most sufferers are well into or beyond their reproductive years and so will have borne children before the disease 'catches up' with them.

The former question, though, regarding the genetic coding for bowel cancer, is more challenging. There are several reasons for this. In looking at the patterns and distribution of bowel cancer in families, it can be fairly difficult to distinguish between genetic and environmental causes. In a study carried out at St Mark's Hospital, London in 1976, it was observed that one-quarter of the patients with colorectal cancer had at least one other member of their family with the same condition. Is this sufficient evidence that there is a genetic cause or predisposition to bowel cancer in such families? The answer to this question must be 'no', since we know that the environment for members of the same families (such as diet and other aspects of life-style) are bound to be similar. So, without very specific ways of looking at and understanding what the genes control and do, it is difficult to separate genetic from environmental factors. This, of course, is true for many diseases. One way around this problem is to describe patterns of disease suggesting a family predisposition as evidence of the **familial** (as opposed to genetic) nature of the disease. Whether this is due to genetic susceptibility or environmental conditioning, or both, is often a difficult question to answer with certainty.

There are several situations in which genetic predisposition appears likely. Many families have now been observed in which the risk of bowel cancer (and other cancers such as breast, ovarian, and uterine) is increased markedly. Such 'cancer families' are presumed to have genes which, when passed on to children, predispose them to the risk of the development of these cancers. The average age of onset of bowel cancer in such patients (late 40s) is about 20 years earlier than is usual for bowel cancer, perhaps suggesting that environmental factors are less important or perhaps 'work quicker' in these people.

The task of finding the genes responsible for the inherited risk of bowel cancer, whether in familial adenomatous polyposis (FAP) or the other forms of 'family cancer', is an immense one: finding a needle in a haystack looks easy in comparison! But in the past few years, the gene responsible for FAP was localized to a particular area of one of our chromosomes, the 'blueprints' for the development and maintenance of the human body, to be found in every one of our cells; within the past year the gene has been located precisely, allowing us now to work out exactly what the gene does. By finding out its precise mode of action, it might be possible to counteract it, thus preventing the adenomas from developing and hence preventing cancer without surgery. And if it's possible for FAP, it may become possible in other forms of inherited cancer risk. At the moment this is all in the future; but experience so far strongly suggests that these speculations will become reality in the not too distant future.

ARE THERE ANY OTHER CAUSATIVE FACTORS IN BOWEL CANCER?

Social, occupational, and economic factors

Whereas most diseases which afflict humankind are a bigger problem for the poor than the rich, bowel cancer appears to be an exception. On an international basis, it is clearly a disease of the developed, industrialized countries which enjoy, on average, a higher material standard of living. Within these countries, however, there is a great variation of social and economic status, and it would be of interest to know whether this maldistribution of wealth affects the distribution of bowel cancer throughout the populations within countries. It is likely that these factors work through their effect on diet, as discussed earlier.

Also, there is evidence that the outcome of treatment of cancer is associated with social and economic status: in general, better survival rates are enjoyed by the rich, and this has been found specifically for rectal cancer as well.

Conditions which predispose to bowel cancer

Besides the hereditary conditions that predispose to bowel cancer, a disparate range of other conditions should be considered.

Inflammatory diseases of the bowel

Patients with long-standing, extensive inflammatory disease of the bowel are known to be at increased risk for bowel cancer although the reasons for this are not known. These diseases are detailed below.

Ulcerative colitis   Ulcerative colitis is a chronic disease of the large bowel in which the inner lining undergoes ulceration (small erosions) and inflammation. This results in recurring symptoms of pain, diarrhoea, and bleeding. Patients with long-standing severe disease are at increased risk to develop cancer—about 10 times that of people with 'normal' bowels, but the reason for this is unknown.

Crohn's disease   Crohn's disease of the colon is the other important inflammatory disease of the large bowel. Crohn's disease may affect the entire gastrointestinal tract (most commonly the small bowel) and is associated with an increased risk of cancer of the large bowel (probably about twice that of the 'normal' population).

Previous bowel cancer

Patients who have been treated for one bowel cancer may be at increased risk for developing a second: probably about two or three times that of those who have not had bowel cancer. This is one of the reasons why such patients are often followed up by regular examinations in an attempt to diagnose new cancers as early as possible.

Previous surgery

Uterosigmoidostomy   In the past, some patients whose bladder needed to be removed completely, usually for cancer, had their urine drained into the colon (by attaching the ureters draining the urine from the kidneys) so that they passed urine with their bowel motions. It became apparent that this placed them at higher than average risk to develop bowel cancer at the site of the connection between the ureter and the bowel, so this technique is now no longer used.

Gall bladder surgery?   There has been some discussion in recent years about the possibility that removal of the gall bladder (cholecystectomy) predisposes to bowel cancer, based on the assumption that this might increase the flow of bile acids into the bowel. This relationship is difficult to study, but the majority conclusion at the moment is that cholecyst-ectomy does not predispose to bowel cancer.

Stomach surgery? Similar discussion has occurred in relation to stomach surgery in patients suffering from a peptic ulcer. There appears to be an increased occurrence of bowel cancer in those who have undergone such surgery. Whether this is due to changes in the production of bile acids, to changes in the bowel bacteria which break down bile acids to produce the 'cancer promoters' discussed earlier (see p. 45), or to some other effect is not known.

SO WHO *DOES* GET BOWEL CANCER?

Common thoughts, and, indeed, voiced questions, in cancer patients and their relatives are: 'Why me?', or, 'Why us?' 'What have I done to deserve this?' Usually the 'off-the-cuff' medical answer is: 'Well, it's just one of those things,' or 'It's not your fault', or 'We don't know, but the important thing now is to get on with treatment so that we can get you back to health.' With more thought it is usually possible to give more helpful answers than these. With all the foregoing evidence in mind, let us look at the whole population and try to pick out any groups known to be at particular risk for bowel cancer.

What effect does our age have on bowel cancer risk?

Despite decades of effort to work out factors which put an individual at increased risk for bowel cancer, and despite all the evidence discussed earlier indicating that some populations are at greater risk than others, when it comes down to *individual* risk, the most important predictor remains a rather simple one—a person's age. The older we get, the higher our chances of getting bowel cancer. It is very rare before the age of 40: less than 3 per cent of all cases in England and Wales occur below that age. The average age of diagnosis is about 70 years. The rate of occurrence rises consistently with age; its rate of rise is similar to the rate of rise of other cancers of the lining tissues of the body which are exposed to cancer-causing agents (e.g. smoke and lung cancer, ultraviolet light and skin cancer). This pattern is consistent with theories of dietary or faecal cancer-causing substances, which take a relatively long time to exert their effect. A corollary of this theory is that cases which occur before the fifth decade of life (40s) are less likely to be due primarily to dietary/environmental factors, and therefore that genetic influences may be relatively more important in cases arising at a younger age. Indeed, this fits with the observations that patients from high-risk 'cancer-prone' families tend to get their cancers at a younger age.

Are men or women at greater risk?

Although both sexes are at very similar risk for large bowel cancer, there are differences which may prove important in our understanding of the causes of the disease. In most countries, cancer of the rectum is slightly more common in men than women, whereas cancer of the colon is overall slightly more common in women than men. These differences, however, are affected by age. Beyond the age of 65, there are more cases of both colon and rectal cancer in women. However, this is because women live about six years longer than men in most countries (i.e. there are more old women than old men). When the incidence *rate* is considered (to cancel out the effect of more older women), both colon and rectal cancer are more common in men than women *after the age of 65*. One explanation for this might be that men, for some reason, become progressively more exposed to the cancer-causing agent(s) than women in later years, or that the decrease in male hormones which perhaps protect men slightly in the earlier years leave them relatively more susceptible as the years pass on. At the moment there is no hard evidence in this area.

How important is a family history of bowel cancer?

We discussed this earlier, and it is easy to get it out of proportion, so we should emphasize that, although a history of bowel cancer in the family appears to be relevant for some patients, the great majority of cases appear to be 'sporadic', that is, they are not the result of an apparent inherited cause or pattern. This subject is discussed in greater detail in later sections, see pp. 67 and 83.

What about social, occupational, and economic factors?

As discussed earlier, these factors are important. An illustration of their likely effect within one country, Finland, is a clear example. In Finland, a country of relatively high incidence, farmers have only 60 per cent of the expected rate of colon cancers, whereas managerial employees have about 25 per cent more cases than the national average; self-employed persons (other than farmers) had 67 per cent more bowel cancer than expected. Amongst those who get bowel cancer, wealth appears to be an advantage; studies carried out in the UK have shown that the upper classes are more likely to survive their cancers.

SUMMARY

Bowel cancer is predominantly a disease of industrialized Western countries, though it is beginning to make an appearance in the 'developing' countries of the world. There is much circumstantial evidence to suggest that this pattern is related to the life-style of the affluent countries, and in particular the refined diet that has resulted from industrialization of food production. Genetic predisposition and the role of predisposing inflammatory diseases are areas of importance as an understanding of their mechanisms of action may help us to understand the disease process more clearly, while recognition of those at risk due to these factors may allow us to prevent cancer in these people. More of this later (see p. 66).

4
Prevention and screening in bowel cancer

'An ounce of prevention is worth a pound of cure' is the sort of saying which seems to ooze manifest good sense. It's no surprise to hear politicians saying that prevention is to play a much greater part in health care in the future: it sounds good and offers hope for the future. But for the moment, in cancer at least, preventive medicine is in its infancy; it will take some time to develop cancer prevention to the stage that it has reached in infectious diseases, such as tuberculosis, smallpox, and the childhood infections. We have seen already that treatment of bowel cancer, once it has reached the stage at which symptoms develop, is successful in only a proportion of patients; so efforts to **prevent** the disease or to detect it earlier by **screening**, in the hope that earlier treatment will improve the patient's chances of cure, are two areas which deserve (and are receiving) the vigorous attention of the research community.

The terms 'prevention' and 'screening' are sometimes used rather loosely. In the case of bowel cancer, strictly, 'prevention' should be used to refer to prevention of the whole train of events from the earliest cellular changes that lead to adenoma formation and on to invasive cancer—this is what we call **primary prevention. Secondary prevention** has the same important practical outcome, the prevention of cancer, but involves the lesser target of detecting and treating people who have benign adenomas and removing these on the assumption that cancer cannot form except from adenomas. **Screening** is something different again. This is the detection of disease in people free of any symptoms of that disease. In other words, in screening we are not aiming to prevent the disease itself, but to prevent the disease from doing so much harm by earlier diagnosis and treatment. Secondary prevention and screening sometimes overlap as we will see shortly.

Primary prevention works best if we have a complete understanding of the causes of a disease and the ways in which we can intervene to separate cause from its effect. Knowing that the tubercle bacillus causes tuberculosis, and that pasteurizing kills this germ, is a classical form of primary prevention. Childhood immunization programmes are a further example. Even though we don't know exactly how cigarette smoke induces lung cancer, we aim at primary prevention by encouraging people to stop smoking. Screening well women by taking cervical smears, is a form of secondary prevention in that it aims to identify women with benign changes in the cervix which herald the development of cancer. By finding such women and removing the areas of benign change, cancer is effectively prevented.

So far so good. But as with all medical measures there is often a 'down side'. Immunization of thousands of infants to prevent measles, whooping cough, etc., prevents much misery and saves lives, but at the very small (in terms of numbers affected) risk of brain damaged children. For those adversely affected by immunization in this way, any benefit from primary prevention of the target disease pales into insignificance. On a lesser level, those who are identified as having high blood pressure, and who may be at a lower risk of heart attacks or strokes by taking medication to treat it, are at some risk of side-effects from those drugs. In offering any preventive measure, therefore, the doctors involved have a responsibility to recognize the adverse effects, to inform those offered the measure of those effects, and to do what they can to minimize them.

PRIMARY PREVENTION

Let's look at primary prevention as it might be applied to bowel cancer. The first major problem that we encounter is our relative lack of knowledge of the steps in the development of the disease at a cellular level. How can we prevent something when we don't know what exactly we are preventing? We know that bowel cancer, and perhaps all cancers, develop through changes in the genes inside our cells, and that the genetic changes which lead to cancer alter the ways in which cells grow and multiply. If we are to intervene to prevent the cellular changes that lead to cancer, therefore, we have to know what can cause the genes to become abnormal. The precise identity of the gene that is abnormal in familial adenomatous polyposis (FAP) has been discovered recently. Next, the function of the gene must be determined, and ways of counteracting that function may be developed. It may well be that this genetic abnormality plays a part in the evolution of bowel cancer in others besides those afflicted with FAP.

For the moment, however, the nearest we can get to **primary** prevention in the genetic conditions which predispose to bowel cancer, is to try to identify involved families and to offer genetic counselling and prenatal diagnosis to those at risk. It may become possible to offer some 'antidote' to the product of the FAP gene some time in the future.

Primary prevention in bowel cancer might also be achieved by preventing the action of those agents which may cause genetic changes in those born with 'normal' genes. As discussed in Chapter 3 (see pp. 40–6) there is much evidence and speculation on the role of a series of dietary factors which might play a part in the causation of bowel cancer, and studies are taking place to see whether alteration of dietary intake of some of these factors might diminish the risk of bowel cancer. People's dietary habits, evolved and ingrained through their lifetimes, are difficult to record for the purposes of research and difficult to change for possible cancer prevention. It is likely that in order to produce a sufficient change in diet to produce a major effect on bowel cancer risk, we would have to 'eat African', in other words, take on the whole dietary approach of a low-bowel cancer incidence area. Studies are in progress of the simple addition of possible protective agents (see Chapter 3, p. 46), such as calcium salts, with no other dietary change, but even simple measures like this are difficult to evaluate in large populations.

SECONDARY PREVENTION AND SCREENING

For the moment, therefore, the greatest research effort in bowel cancer prevention is going into secondary prevention and screening—the detection and treatment of those with non-symptomatic adenomas or small cancers—to see whether this might decrease the risk from bowel cancer. We could look at screening as it affects the individual's risk, but much more effort has gone into trying to decide whether, if screening were to be taken up as a public health measure (as with immunization), it would have an effect on the population-wide consequences of the target disease. In this description we will concentrate on this approach.

Screening—early diagnosis in asymptomatic people

There is good evidence from countries that run efficient cervix cancer screening programmes, that the death rate from this disease can be cut dramatically. Iceland has played a leading role in the implementation of cervical cancer screening—it and the other Nordic countries are particularly efficient in this regard, and have reaped the reward accordingly. A national breast cancer screening programme was implemented in the UK when the Department of Health became satisfied with the evidence from research trials that this would have a sufficient effect on the death rate for this condition. There is no national UK screening programme for bowel cancer at the present time, although in some parts of the country tests are being offered as part of research studies to find out how useful screening might be. In other countries such as West Germany and to a lesser degree the US and Canada, screening tests for bowel cancer are offered on a regular basis by doctors who consider that it is useful for their patients.

What would bowel cancer screening involve for the individual?

The essence of bowel cancer screening is the application of a simple, safe, cheap test (a faecal occult, i.e. hidden, or invisible, blood test most commonly), upon the result of which will depend whether people go on to a second, more complex and expensive test (colonoscopy or barium enema X-ray) which should decide with great precision whether bowel cancer or adenomas are present. There are several ways to do this, but the simplest and most practical at the moment is to search for hidden blood in the bowel motion. This exploits the fact that most bowel cancers bleed slightly: so slightly that it cannot be seen by the naked eye. There are now several methods available which can detect such blood but the best studied test, Haemoccult, involves applying chemicals to a sample of stool: if a blue coloration appears on the test card, the test is positive.

The 'Haemoccult' test—how is it done?

Prior to performing the test, the subject may be asked to restrict the diet, avoiding large quantities of Vitamin C, red meat, and certain vegetables such as turnips and horseradish: any of these can affect the outcome of the test. This is advised for two days prior to the testing and during the three days of the testing.

The patient is instructed to obtain two pea-sized samples of stool from a bowel motion, using a small disposable cardboard spatula. These are then placed on a test card, which is closed up and delivered to the doctor's surgery or to a laboratory; a drop of hydrogen peroxide is added to the sample which is watched during the next minute for a blue colour change. The chemical reaction is based on the fact that guaiac, a *colour-less* plant gum resin, is transformed into a quinone, a *blue* compound, in the presence of peroxide (from the dropper) and a peroxidase enzyme. Because the haemoglobin (the iron-containing molecule within red blood cells) has peroxidase properties, its presence in the stool triggers the reaction thus producing the tell-tale blue colour. Without peroxidase (or the haemoglobin of red blood cells) the reaction does not occur, there is no colour change and the test is interpreted as negative. Those with a positive result are recommended to undergo further tests (see p. 80).

Unfortunately faecal occult blood tests cannot distinguish between blood shed from cancers and that from problems such as piles. Hidden blood from other causes in the absence of symptoms is not likely to be of clinical importance—another way of saying that nothing need be done. Like all tests in medicine, it is far from perfect.

What happens after the Haemoccult test?

For all the reasons stated above, a firm diagnosis cannot be made on the basis of the Haemoccult test alone, as it is a *screening test*, not a *diagnostic* or *confirmatory test*. In fact only about one in ten *positive* **tests in individuals in the 45–75 age group** (those who might be considered for mass screening) **would be found on confirmatory testing to have a bowel cancer**. On the other hand a negative test implies that the probability of a missed cancer (false negative) is about 1 in 2000. While these results are clearly imperfect, the screening test is fairly effective at identifying people at significantly higher (or lower risk) than the average (untested) population. A positive test increases the likelihood of bowel cancer in an asymptomatic apparently well person by about 40 times, while a negative test reduces that same likelihood by a factor of about 4 times.

While a negative test can be reassuring for the person, it does not, of course, rule out the possibility of bowel cancer becoming apparent in the future. Therefore, all such patients must be warned not to ignore any symptoms which might develop. If that were to happen, the dangers of false reassurance might be quite serious. If a mass screening programme were to become established, all eligible subjects would be encouraged to attend regularly at intervals of two years or so to try to pick up any cancers which might develop in the future.

Subjects who have a positive test should be reviewed by their family doctor to establish that the test was carried out correctly and that further investigation is appropriate. If appropriate, a more definitive test is offered to the patient. This may be another faecal occult blood test under more stringent testing conditions, namely a restricted diet if that wasn't recommended or adhered to the first time around. Instead of that, or after a repeat positive test, the next step is either a colonscopy or a barium enema X-ray (and flexible sigmoidoscopy, if possible). In general, a colonoscopy is probably better than the X-ray since it can detect smaller tumours and allows immediate biopsy or removal of any abnormalities seen.

General issues in screening

So the test itself is simple to perform and to interpret, and the further investigations resulting from a positive test are quite straightforward. However, before recommending a mass screening programme (whereby everyone in the population of the appropriate sex and age is offered a particular screening test), it is important to establish that the potential benefits of such a programme will outweigh any potential harm, and that the net benefits are worth the hardships and costs. This can be very difficult to prove, largely because the objective measurement of the benefits and harms of medical interventions is very difficult. Such methods are still in the early stages of development. Furthermore, to evaluate such outcomes accurately and with enough precision takes very large, long and expensive research projects. Even then, the results can be difficult to analyse and may be open to several interpretations. In other words, the decision to implement screening as a routine procedure is almost always a controversial and hotly debated topic, which usually continues long after the political decision is made. For instance, doctors in the UK continue to argue over the usefulness of breast cancer screening even though it is now part of UK National Health Service provision, while cervical cancer screening, which is more widely accepted as useful, is diminished in its effect in the UK by poor administration.

How should we evaluate screening in a particular disease, then? There are several critical questions which must be answered.

Is the disease a big enough problem to warrant screening?

This, of course, begs the question what is 'big enough' and relative to what? Ideally, all diseases which pose a threat to humans are big enough problems to warrant improved diagnosis and treatment. But in the political and economic realities of our time, the need to define priorities in health care increasingly demands that we evaluate and compare their consequences and costs. Few would dispute that bowel cancer, the second commonest cancer killer in the Western world, is a major health problem and warrants significant efforts to reduce its mortality and morbidity.

Does earlier diagnosis—before the onset of symptoms—help?

This is the most important question to be answered and it is the most difficult. It's no good just showing that available screening tests can detect cancer in apparently healthy people. Nor even is it enough to show that patients whose cancer is detected by screening live longer after diagnosis than those treated after they have symptoms. Both of these could be true if the test merely makes the diagnosis earlier in time but does not alter the time of death due to the disease. Such a screening test *would only lengthen the period during which one was aware of the presence of a disease*, but it would not add years to one's life. A test that merely achieved this would clearly be detrimental. Another important problem in the evaluation of screening tests for fatal diseases is that any screening test tends to detect those individuals with *less aggressive* disease: those in whom the disease has been so aggressive that it has led to death rapidly are not around to be tested. Screening can be compared to a torpedo passing through a convoy of ships; just as the torpedo tends to hit the longer ships, so screening tends to select out those with longer lasting, i.e. less aggressive, disease. So if we are not careful, we may look at the outcome of treatment in a group of patients who have had their disease detected by screening, and be impressed erroneously by the good results achieved by treatment of what is in fact an unrepresentative selection of cancer patients. One way to show whether a screening test actually improves the outcome is to carry out a so-called randomized controlled trial, to compare the results of treatment for that disease when detected in a screened population compared to the results in an unscreened population. In such a study, a large population is randomly divided into two halves, equivalent in all respects except that one group is offered screening and the other is not. The death rate for the disease and any other relevant statistics are then compared at, say, 5 and 10 years from the beginning of the study. Trials like this are under way in several countries to answer these difficult questions about the usefulness of bowel cancer screening.

Is the test accurate enough?

Inaccurate tests can have serious consequences. When a test is used to detect cancer there are two possible test results (positive and negative), two possible cancer statuses (cancer present or absent), and four possible combinations of results and cancer status:

Table 5. The four possible combinations of results and cancer status

	Cancer present	Cancer absent
Test positive	1. **True** positive	2. **False** positive
Test negative	3. **False** negative	4. **True** negative

1. **A true positive test**—the test result is **positive** in a person who does have cancer. This is the result (and the patient) which every screening programme is trying to find. The $64 000 question is whether finding such a patient gives them a better chance of benefiting from treatment than if they had not been identified until after symptoms appeared.

2. **A false positive test**—when the test result is positive in a person who does not have cancer. Such a person can hardly benefit from such a result and suffers, unfortunately, as the innocent victim of unnecessary worry and anxiety as well as the inconvenience and discomfort of further tests. In the end, of course, they are rewarded with the good news that all is well. But that is little compensation; it would have been better had it been a true negative in the first place.

About 2 per cent (1 in 50) of people who *do not* have bowel cancer will have a *false positive* Haemoccult test, because:

- Blood in the stool may originate from anywhere along the digestive tract, from the mouth to the anus. Therefore blood from any site (e.g. bleeding gums or an inflamed lining of the stomach as occurs in gastritis or an ulcer) may result in a positive test.
- A small amount of bleeding occurs normally in the human digestive tract, even if there are no identifiable pathological conditions. This may occur from the normal shedding and replacement of the mucosa (lining) of the stomach or bowels, or from minor irritations or scratches from food or other swallowed objects.
- Some foods may themselves cause a positive reaction. This may occur from the ingestion of meats which contain the red blood cells

of animals (especially undercooked beef or lamb); the test does not distinguish human blood from other sources. Similarly, certain vegetables, such as turnips and horseradish, contain 'pseudo-peroxidase', which can cause a positive reaction.

3. A false negative test—when the test result is negative in a person who does have cancer. Some people consider this to be the worst kind of error in a screening programme, because it means that the test has failed that one individual in the main aim of the programme—to detect a cancer which is there at the time of the screening. The main danger for a person who has a false negative test is the development of a false sense of security about the disease screened for; so that if and when symptoms do develop (from the cancer which was missed), the appropriate action will not be taken. In fact, there is no evidence that this is the case; it is at least as possible that the heightened awareness of the disease in someone who has already participated in a screening programme would make them more likely to recognize and respond to symptoms when they appear.

About one in four people who *have* cancer of the bowel will have a *false negative* Haemoccult test, for one of various reasons:

- Bleeding from tumours is not constant; it is intermittent, in other words, there may not be enough blood in the stool to produce a positive test at the time the test is done. To minimize this problem, the test is repeated on three bowel motions over three days. Increasing the number of days of testing to six further reduces the chance for a false negative result from about 25 per cent to about 10 per cent.
- Only a small sample of faeces is taken at any one time; if blood is not evenly distributed throughout the stool, then none may be included in the sample.
- The presence of large amounts of Vitamin C in the stool may interfere with the chemical reaction and produce a false negative result.
- If the test is not interpreted within 3 or 4 days of collecting the specimen, there is an increasing probability that a false negative test will occur due to drying out and degradation of the chemicals involved in the test.
- Test design or manufacturing imperfections.

4. A true negative test—when the result is negative in a person who does not have cancer. This is the most common test result in all cancer screening programmes. At the time the test is performed it cannot be assumed that a negative result is a *true* negative, though the chance that

it is a *false* negative is only about 1 : 2000. A more important risk is that the person told that their test was negative may acquire a long-term false sense of security and ignore future symptoms when a cancer develops at a later time.

It is probably impossible to design any screening test which is perfect; adjustments can be made to reduce the number of false positives, but this invariably increases the number of false negatives, so a trade-off and compromise between the two has to be reached at all times.

It is important to keep in mind that a screening test is not the same as a definitive diagnostic test. A screening test is just that—a screen to divide apparently well people into two groups—those very unlikely to have the disease in question and those who are much more likely to have it. The next step in all screening programmes is to apply a more accurate (and usually more uncomfortable and expensive) test to establish a more definitive diagnosis. In breast screening, the first test is the mammogram; the definitive diagnostic test is the breast biopsy—a small surgical procedure to get a sample of the lump for analysis under a microscope. In bowel cancer screening, the first test is a simple test on the stool to look for hidden blood; the definitive test is either a barium enema X-ray or, preferably, to look inside the bowel directly using a colonoscope.

Is the test acceptable to people?

The simplest, cheapest, most technically precise test in the world will be of little use if the population to be offered screening does not find the test generally acceptable. This is known as 'compliance', and has varied between 15 and 50 + per cent in bowel cancer screening studies using faecal occult blood tests. Different ways of collecting the stool sample and of applying the chemicals to detect blood have been tried but seem not to affect compliance much. Members of the general public are not very aware of bowel cancer, so perhaps it is not surprising that they are often slow to accept the chance to collect stool specimens! It may be, if the randomized trials of screening suggest that it has a useful effect, that public awareness and acceptance will increase.

Are the subsequent tests and treatments acceptable?

This is an important question: having defined a group for further invest-igation by faecal occult blood screening, we have to be happy that the further investigations (colonoscopy or X-ray) and treatment, if cancer is confirmed, are acceptable to the public. In fact, colonoscopy is a fairly straightforward procedure which does not normally require admission to hospital and which most patients do not find difficult to tolerate. There is a small risk of injury, and a minute risk of death as a result, associated with colonoscopy. Again this is something that those examining the usefulness of bowel cancer screening must be aware of, because those suffering such injuries are unlikely to have a cancer anyway, so the net benefit for them is very negative. If adenomas or a very small cancer are found, it is often possible to treat it via the colonoscope at the same sitting. Larger cancers will require a major operation to remove them, but as the majority of such procedures are routine, they do not of themselves present a great threat to those undergoing them.

Do the overall benefits to the community sufficiently outweigh the harms and costs to make the establishment of a screening programme worthwhile?

In the end we have to balance any positive benefit for the populace against the negative consequences—the anxiety for all those who have a positive faecal occult blood test yet turn out to have nothing wrong, the few who will be injured by the colonoscopy, and the financial cost, the resources that have been put into the screening programme, and which might have been more usefully spent on hip replacements, psychiatric nurses, etc. Some politicians might also rather discreetly point out the cost to the Exchequer of support for all the pensionable people who may live longer and drain state resources! All these costs are difficult to quantify, making it almost impossible to define ahead of time the possible cost/benefit ratio for bowel cancer screening.

Other methods of mass screening

So far, we have concentrated on the use of the Haemoccult test, and have discussed all the big issues relating to bowel cancer screening as if this were the only method available; in fact, although they haven't been investigated anywhere nearly as thoroughly as Haemoccult, there are other tests and methods that deserve mention.

Other faecal occult blood tests

Other tests have been developed which use the same chemical test as Haemoccult: some of these are offered in the same way, as cards upon which stool is collected. Others require the user to wipe their bottom with 'magic toilet paper'—either a simple tissue onto which the chemicals can be sprayed after use, or paper into which some of the chemicals have been impregnated, requiring peroxide to be dripped on after use. A novel approach is to impregnate a piece of paper with the test chemicals, and instead of using it as toilet paper, drop it into the toilet bowl after the stool has been passed in the hope that any blood in the stool will seep out into the water and thereby become available to cause a colour change in the test paper. The limited testing of these various methods has looked at chemical efficiency in cancer detection and at their acceptability relative to Haemoccult, but none has stood out as being superior; indeed, one or two have been shown to be very poor alternatives in their present form, either due to high false positive or false negative rates.

Other faecal occult blood tests use different chemical means for detecting blood. HaemoQuant is one such test, which can quantify the amount of blood present; as the amount might give a clue to the origin of the blood, this is seen by some as a technical advantage. The test is more complicated to perform and rather more expensive than Haemoccult, so it is not seen as a potential mass screening test. Another sort of occult blood test exploits the new technology of monoclonal antibodies (see p. 137). These tests, known as immunoassays, have the theoretical advantage of being able to detect human blood only, so decreasing the false positive rate, and with it the anxiety and cost associated with false positive results. So far, however, these tests have not proven themselves to be more discriminating than Haemoccult.

Faecal tumour product tests

It ought to be possible to detect substances other than blood shed into the bowel motions. Theoretically cancer cells shed into the stool should contain proteins which only occur in cancer cells, or at least in larger amounts than in normal cells. Carcinoembryonic antigen (CEA, see p. 141) is one such substance, but attempts to use this as a 'stool marker' have failed on technical grounds so far. The chemically different mucus produced by cancer cells is another possible target substance. There is now some evidence that cancer-causing genes, shed into the stool, may be detectable in the faeces. This would certainly be a major leap forward in screening technology.

Tumour markers in the blood

A completely different approach is to look for substances released from tumours into the blood ('tumour markers'). Again, CEA has been investigated—20–30 years ago, when this substance was first discovered, it was seen as the great hope for screening. But it misses a large proportion of early cancers, and may be present in increased amounts in the blood of people with other conditions or with no condition at all! And anyway, the prospect of mass screening using a blood test is seen by many researchers as a more complicated and costly approach than testing the stool.

Endoscopic screening

Yet another approach is the use of endoscopy, direct examination of the bowel lining using flexible 'telescopes'. Mass colonoscopy is a non-starter due to the expense and the risks of injury when performed on very large numbers of people. But the shorter 'flexible sigmoidoscope' might be used as a quick test to examine that part of the bowel most likely to harbour cancers and adenomas, the rectum and sigmoid colon. Again, it has the disadvantage of expense and the expertise required to use the equipment, but studies in the US are beginning to show that this test could be performed perfectly well with limited training by nurses or technicians. This whole area needs to be investigated more thoroughly, and it will be a while yet before we know whether endoscopic screening is likely to be a useful idea.

Selective screening of high risk groups

Use of faecal occult blood testing, or whatever other mass screening test seems appropriate, aims to select from the wider population a smaller group for more detailed scrutiny, based on their higher risk of cancer as suggested by the screening test. Another way to define a smaller group is to look at aspects of the individuals which might place them into a 'high risk group' without the need to subject them to any further test. Let's look at these 'high risk groups'.

Family history and cancer risk

Most people are aware that cancer seems to 'run' in some families; certainly there are such families, as we discussed in Chapter 3 (see p. 46). At its most extreme, this predisposition to develop cancer may be inherited on average by half the offspring of someone carrying the risk. If we just look at the close relatives of anyone who develops bowel cancer, it appears that there is an overall increase in risk amongst them of around two to three times the average population risk. We discussed the matter in detail in Chapter 3, and perhaps that section should be re-read at this stage: suffice to say here that doctors caring for bowel cancer patients are becoming more aware of these family-related risks, and that several clinics have been set up around the country to look specifically at the care of such families, and to counsel those who are anxious that their family may be carrying some increased risk. It is likely that any mass screening programme set up in the future will include an initial questionnaire to pick out those who appear to be members of 'cancer families', and to send some of these directly for colonoscopy, rather than bother with a faecal occult blood test initially. Until we know more about the genetic abnormalities causing this increased risk, we will not be able to advise people very precisely on their familial risk. Till then we have to base our advice on taking careful details of the family pedigree and interpreting what we see rather empirically.

Known conditions of high risk

Besides familial predisposition, there are certain medical conditions which predispose to bowel cancer.

Previous bowel cancer This is the most obvious example. It is partly because people who have had bowel cancer carry a 5 per cent risk of developing a completely new bowel cancer (rather than a recurrence of the previous one) that most surgeons examine patients regularly after surgery. Some perform regular colonoscopy to try to detect adenomas or early cancers.

Inflammatory bowel disease Ulcerative colitis and, to a lesser extent, Crohn's disease can increase an individual's bowel cancer risk. This was discussed in Chapter 3 (see p. 49). As long-standing (i.e. more than 10 years) ulcerative colitis sufferers with extensive involvement of the colon and rectum are at particular risk, they should be picked out for special surveillance. Most doctors would agree that they should be seen every year or two; they should be questioned carefully regarding their symptoms, and biopsies should be taken from the bowel lining, looking for the tell-tale microscopic signs of 'dysplasia', a change in the appearance of the bowel lining cells which may suggest that cancer could develop in the near future, or may even already have occurred elsewhere in the bowel. Complete colonoscopic examination of this patient group, at regular intervals, is practised by many centres looking after colitis patients.

SUMMARY

Bowel cancer prevention, or for the moment, prevention of *death* due to bowel cancer by early detection, is a laudable aim and one into which much research effort is being directed. True prevention will require a more complete understanding of the causative factors for the disease, while success in screening and secondary prevention demands better tests, uptake by those at most risk, and more resources if the current randomized trials show screening to be a worthwhile approach to decreasing the death rate for this common disease.

5

The symptoms of bowel cancer and when to go to the doctor

Most of us tend to think of normal health and disease as being quite clearly separable, but often this is not the case. The onset of the symptoms of bowel cancer is a very good example of how ill health may creep up on us without being very obvious at first. Little wonder that on average there is a delay of about six months between the onset of the symptoms of bowel cancer and seeking out medical advice. The main reason, perhaps, is that the symptoms of bowel cancer tend to mimic those of more common, less serious problems, such as piles.

Before we can say what symptoms should take us along to the doctor, we need to understand a little of how these symptoms might develop, and the grouping together of symptoms that should be taken particularly seriously. The first thing to say, which for anyone blessed with the sort of bowel function that they could set their watch by may come as a surprise, is that there is a great variety and range of normal function between different people. Furthermore, we all get aches, pains, and other symptoms which we blame on our 'stomach' or 'bowel'; for some of us these are a regular, and sometimes very disabling, part of life, though often they are not due to any identifiable and serious underlying cause. One of the aims of this chapter is to provide sensible guidelines about when to consult a doctor about symptoms which may be warnings for serious bowel trouble.

Firstly, we should list the symptoms which may warn of bowel cancer, and then try to define 'normal bowel function' so that we can see how bowel cancer symptoms may develop and differ from our normal pattern.

THE IMPORTANT SYMPTOMS OF BOWEL CANCER

- **Change in bowel habit** (i.e. change in the frequency, and the solidity, or otherwise, of bowel movements);

- Blood and/or mucus with the motions;
- Abdominal pain;
- Tenesmus (a constant feeling of incomplete emptying of the bowel, despite regular bowel movements);
- General symptoms (weight loss, tiredness, loss of appetite, etc.).

WHAT *IS* 'NORMAL BOWEL FUNCTION'?

A survey of a random sample of south Londoners aged 55 years and older revealed a remarkable variation in beliefs and attitudes about the bowels. Like all surveys, its results cannot be taken as certain truth, but it does illustrate the range of function that different people accept as normal, and therefore may help us to know what to think about our own bowel habit. The results of the survey are shown in Table 6. Men reported moving their bowels more often than women; two-thirds of the men and just over half of the women moved their bowels once daily. About one-fifth of men and one-tenth of women did not have motions every day. A large majority of both sexes reported that their bowel patterns were regular; 95 per cent of men and 86 per cent of women could predict their frequency of bowel actions.

Table 6. Frequency of bowel movements among south Londoners aged 55 and over

Frequency of bowel movements	Males	Females
Once daily	67%	56%
Less than once daily	18%	8%
More than once daily	21%	12%
No predictable frequency	5%	14%

In the survey, most of the respondents were satisfied by their bowel frequency, only 11 per cent felt that their bowels did not open often enough and only 3 per cent thought that their bowels opened too frequently. For about one in seven respondents, satisfactory results were achieved after some effort. They habitually used something to keep their bowels regular: usually several methods. Two-thirds used 'over the counter' laxatives and over half deliberately used vegetables and fruit and/or supplemented their diets with bran to improve their bowel function. Of those who used such aids, the majority had been using them for 5 years or more.

These figures show that bowel habits can vary widely and why it is not possible or useful to try to define too narrowly what is 'normal', so what should we consider as abnormal function worthy of concern and consultation with a doctor?

What are the differences between 'normal' bowel function and the symptoms of bowel cancer?

The presence of bowel cancer may make itself known in several ways, depending on its location in the bowel and its state of advance. Perhaps the best way to understand the symptoms that may develop is to apply what we have already discussed about the anatomy and function of the bowel. The bowel is a hollow tube containing faeces which is liquid as it enters the caecum, and gradually thickens as its water is absorbed while it makes its way to the rectum. If a growth from the inner lining of that tube gradually enlarges, what trouble can it cause to warn of its presence? There are two main **local effects** of the tumour that may cause symptoms which should engage our attention:

- It can shed **blood** or **mucus** into the faeces; this would result in an **altered appearance and consistency** of the stool.
- It can **narrow the bowel** as the tumour gets bigger; this might result in a **change in stool size, frequency and consistency,** and/or **discomfort or cramping pain** due to the stronger contractions of the bowel needed to push faeces through the narrower channel.

A bowel tumour may also have general effects:

- There may be symptoms due to anaemia, such as **tiredness** and **lethargy.**
- There may be **weight loss** and **loss of appetite,** frequent effects of cancers at any site in the body.

Although there are no set patterns, the local effects may vary in their intensity depending on the position of the tumour in the bowel.

Cancer of the right colon (caecum and ascending colon)

Cancers arising in this region tend to cause symptoms later than tumours further downstream. **Blood** or **mucus** shed into the right colon usually becomes mixed in with the stool and altered by bacterial action by the time it is emptied from the rectum, so obvious blood may not be seen in the motion. If there is a significant loss, blood partially degraded by bacteria may darken the stool, perhaps making it maroon-coloured or even darker. Most commonly, there is no obvious change in the appearance of the motions and the only way to tell whether blood is being lost in the stools is to check for anaemia with a simple blood examination, or to check the stool with a chemical test for occult (hidden) blood. **Tiredness** due to chronic blood loss may be the first symptom of right-sided colon cancer. If unexplained anaemia is found in a person over the age of 40, the possibility of colon cancer should be kept in mind.

Change in bowel habit may be minimal or absent in right-sided colon cancer. This is most likely due to the liquid nature of the faeces in this part of the colon, which allows it to find its way through a narrowed channel. It usually takes a large mass in the caecum or right colon to cause any impediment to the flow of faeces. Thus the tumour's presence may go unnoticed for some time.

Sometimes, and in the absence of any other symptoms, a right-sided cancer can be felt by the patient through the front of the abdomen as a moveable **lump**.

Cancer of the sigmoid colon and rectum

Bleeding from the back passage is the most common symptom of cancer of the sigmoid colon and rectum—the lowest parts of the large bowel. The blood may be well mixed within the stool or, especially in low-lying tumours, may appear as streaks on the surface of the stool, identical to the pattern seen with piles.

Change of bowel habit is a prominent symptom. The bowel loses its normal timetable, with periods of constipation alternating with diarrhoea. Diarrhoea occurs because solid stool is prevented from passing onwards while liquid is able to get through. Narrowing of the sigmoid colon, in particular, is more likely to cause abdominal **cramping pain**. Later the bowel can become completely blocked, causing severe pains, reminiscent of childbirth to female patients, distension of the abdomen and, eventually, vomiting.

An important symptom of rectal cancer is **tenesmus**, the constant feeling of a full rectum. The brain interprets the presence of a tumour mass as stool but, of course, it cannot be passed. This feeling causes frequent visits to the toilet, when straining may only produce some bloody mucus.

A more constant pain in the back or sacral area, not related to bowel motions, can result from the invasion of other structures outside the rectum. This is a later symptom and usually signifies more advanced disease.

Cancer of the transverse and left colon
Tumours in this part of the bowel, lying between the two areas described above, may cause symptoms which overlap these two symptom patterns.

Rarer symptoms of bowel cancer, due to advanced tumours spreading outside the bowel, include:

- **Pain on passing urine**, perhaps with **air or small particles of stool** (looking like tea leaves) **in the urine**. These symptoms can be due to tumour invading the bladder, followed by leakage of stool into the urine stored within it.
- **Passage of stool through the vagina**. This may be due to a tumour in the rectum invading the back of the vagina.

Both symptoms are very distressing, and it might be thought that such problems could only be due to cancer. But it should be pointed out that they can also be due to other, non-malignant bowel conditions.

WHEN SHOULD YOU GO TO THE DOCTOR?

The south London survey mentioned earlier showed that one-third of the respondents had consulted a doctor about their bowels at least once at some time prior to receiving the questionnaire, and nearly half of those aged 65-74 had done so. The commonest reasons for consulting a doctor were, in descending order, constipation, pain, bleeding, diarrhoea, and piles. These were, by design of the survey, people *without* cancer, so the investigation of their symptoms did not lead to a diagnosis of bowel cancer.

As any of these symptoms can be due to less sinister conditions, there is a tendency for many of us to put off 'bothering' the doctor. It is little wonder that, on average, it takes six months for people to become sufficiently concerned by their symptoms to get round to seeking advice.

What, then, *are* the symptoms which justify a visit to the doctor, and how long should they be present before the time comes to ring up the surgery and make the appointment?

1. **Bleeding.** Blood passed from the bowel, especially if mixed with the stool or if dark in colour, should be a signal to see the doctor. Although blood seen only on the toilet paper, or brighter in colour, are less worrying symptoms, it is nevertheless best to be checked out, especially amongst those beyond, say, 50 years of age.

2. **Change in bowel habit.** This important symptom may be only minimal in extent: someone with a long-standing habit of passing one bowel action each morning may find that they have to make a second visit before leaving for work. For others the change may be more obvious. In any case, an unexplained change going on for more than a couple of weeks needs attention.

3. **Pain.** Lots of us get abdominal pains, and in most of us it is not an indication of cancer. But cramping pain, perhaps associated with other symptoms, may be due to a constricting growth in the bowel— when in doubt, check it out.

4. **Tenesmus.** As explained above, a constant feeling of incomplete emptying of the rectum is an important symptom of rectal cancer. If this symptom is present, it should take us to our doctor at an early stage.

In summary, then, the symptoms of bowel cancer may creep up insidiously, and may seem to be of little consequence at first. The main message is: unexplained bowel symptoms which persist for more than a couple of weeks, especially in the middle-aged and elderly, need to be reported to the doctor. Much better to 'waste' the doctor's time than to waste the chance of early diagnosis of a bowel cancer.

6
Seeking medical help

Deciding to go to the doctor is sometimes very straightforward—an injury, a bad cold, itchy spots, and many other problems are self-evident reasons to seek medical advice. But deciding that bowel symptoms need attention may be more difficult. The subject may be embarrassing to talk about, the patient may feel that the doctor tends to be unsympathetic about such matters, or it may be that the symptoms seem too trifling to bother about. As discussed earlier (see p.70), however, bleeding from the bowel or a change in the regularity of the bowel motions going on for more than a couple of weeks should be regarded as enough to propel us towards our family doctor. So what is likely to happen when we take such symptoms along to the surgery? The previous chapter dealt with the symptoms as they make themselves apparent to the patient before going to the doctor. This chapter deals with the consequences of deciding to make that visit—it describes the situation as the doctor sees it and deals with it.

VISITING THE FAMILY DOCTOR

The family doctor is faced with several tasks:

- to get an accurate picture of the problem from the patient;
- to decide on a group of possible diagnoses, hopefully including the correct one;
- to decide whether he or she can manage the problem, or that the patient should be referred to a specialist;
- if referral seems necessary, to decide which specialist is most appropriate;
- to take any immediate steps needed for the comfort and safety of the patient.

The family doctor, unlike the hospital doctor, is likely to have met the patient before and to know them to some extent. This is very important when it comes to assessing the symptoms that the patient describes.

Having heard about the bleeding (especially if the blood is dark) or about the change of bowel habit, the alarm bell should be ringing—on this story alone the doctor should be coming up with a list of diagnostic possibilities which includes bowel cancer. A good doctor will examine the patient, including feeling inside the rectum with a rubber glove, but even if all appears normal, referral is probably indicated by the patient's story. The problem arises, however, of whether *all* patients with these symptoms should be referred to the hospital. Family doctors see lots of patients with minor 'tummy upsets' and small amounts of bleeding, and referral of every one is unnecessary. Bright bleeding only noticed on the toilet paper (likely to be due to piles), or diarrhoea in more than one household member at the same time (likely to be due to gastroenteritis) can be dealt with, at least initially, by the family doctor. But unless some easy explanation is apparent, especially in the over 50s, referral for consultant examination and investigation is necessary. On average, however, there is a six month delay between onset of symptoms and presentation at the hospital in patients with bowel cancer. This delay, generated by the patient and the family doctor, is partly due to the considerable overlap between the symptoms of bowel cancer and those of harmless conditions such as piles.

Most patients with these symptoms will be referred by the family doctor to a surgeon. Often, however, the diagnosis will be far from obvious, the family doctor simply feeling that there may be something seriously wrong but not knowing what or where; the patient may be vaguely unwell, with weight loss, anaemia, etc., in which case the referral may be to a general physician. If the family doctor feels that a surgical referral is appropriate, ideally this should be to a surgeon with a special interest in colorectal diseases, as they are most likely to be able to offer the widest range of specialist procedures needed to treat the various types and stages of bowel cancer.

REFERRAL TO THE HOSPITAL

Coming quickly to a diagnosis, discussing it with the patient and the family doctor, and deciding on appropriate treatment are the main tasks of the specialist. This section deals only with the task of making the diagnosis, the rest comes later.

History taking

Just as the family doctor needed to hear about the symptoms from the patient, the specialist will want to do the same. Although the letter from the family doctor will have briefly outlined the symptoms, the specialist will ask the patient to tell the story again; this will not only allow the surgeon's diagnostic thoughts to begin to tick over, it will also allow him or her to begin to get to know the patient and their insight into the problem. This will be very important when it comes to discussing the diagnosis and treatment later. When the patient has told their story, the surgeon will ask some 'direct' questions, aimed at making the story clearer, amplifying any areas that seem to require it. He or she will want to know about other health problems, past medical history, about the patient's family and job, etc. By the time the history has been taken, the surgeon should have gained as clearly as possible a picture of the patient and their symptoms; only then will he or she be in a position to begin to come to what is known as a differential diagnosis, a short list of two or three main possible causes of the symptoms. Having got this far the next step is to examine the patient.

Physical examination

Although the surgeon may perform a wide-ranging general examination, he or she will be looking in much more detail at those areas highlighted by the patient's story. Having checked for general signs of anaemia, weight loss, jaundice, etc., he or she will examine the abdomen very carefully. He or she will look at the surface to see if there are any obvious swellings, followed by a gentle examination of the whole surface of the abdomen with the palm of the hand. This may reveal a lump in the line of the bowel, or the liver may be enlarged. Next comes percussion, in which one hand is placed on the abdomen and the middle finger struck sharply with the tip of the other middle finger. This strange performance is used to gauge the degree of solidity of the structures immediately within the abdomen, below the right hand. If the bowel is full of gas a sound like a drum is heard, while if a solid organ, such as an enlarged liver, or an abnormal amount of fluid is present a dull thud will be heard. (This technique is said to have been brought into practice by the medical son of a German wine grower who saw his father tapping on his barrels to check on the amount of wine inside.) Finally the surgeon may feel it necessary to listen to the activity of the bowel with a stethoscope, particularly if the story suggests that there might be a partial obstruction of the bowel.

The next part of the examination is done with the patient lying on their left side with the knees bent up towards the chest; this allows the surgeon to feel and look inside the rectum. In some parts of the world, including much of Europe and North America, this examination is done with the patient lying flat on their front on a special table that bends in the middle at the level of the patient's hips. There are two main parts of this examination:

1. **Digital examination.** This involves the surgeon inserting his or her right index finger into the rectum, suitably protected by a plastic glove. This may be an embarrassing experience for the patient, who may also expect it to be painful. If the patient can relax in these circumstances, the muscles of the anal canal are less likely to resist the surgeon's finger, making the examination less uncomfortable. Having applied a little lubricant jelly to the glove, the surgeon will insert it gently into the lower rectum via the anus. The lining of the bowel can be felt quite easily: if there is a tumour within reach of the finger this will be felt as a firm lump, perhaps with a hollowed-out, ulcerated central area. The rectal wall is normally quite mobile on the underlying tissues, but an advanced cancer which has invaded through the bowel wall to involve tissues outside will feel much less mobile than the surrounding normal bowel. Around 75 per cent of rectal cancers (i.e. 35 per cent of all cancers of the colon and rectum) are within reach of the examining finger. On extracting the finger, the surgeon will examine the glove for tell-tale signs of blood or mucus suggestive of a tumour or other abnormality.

2. **Sigmoidoscopy.** This is direct visual examination of the lining of the bowel using a sigmoidoscope. The usual type of instrument is a rigid metal tube, half an inch in diameter and 12 inches long which can reach to the top of the rectum and just beyond. The tube is hollow and has a glass lens attached at the outer end to allow the surgeon to view through it. Built into the lens attachment is a side tube to allow air to be introduced using a small rubber bulb to inflate the rectum gently, making it easier to examine, and a light source to illuminate the inside of the bowel. Just as with the digital examination, the patient may be anxious at the thought of this examination. Insertion of the instrument through the anus is not painful. As it is advanced along the rectum, and air is introduced into the bowel, the patient may have a feeling of needing to

empty the bowel. Sometimes the air escapes from the rectum around the scope, causing further embarrassment to the patient, though the surgeon knows that this is a regular occurrence in this situation and will hopefully try to allay the patient's feelings. The normal lining of the bowel is a yellowish pink colour; the surface is shiny and the blood vessels within the wall can be seen through the lining. As the scope is advanced the surgeon may see blood or mucus in the bowel, a strongly suspicious sign of a tumour at a higher level. A tumour coming into vision looks very different from the normal lining. It may be a discrete lump or a ring of abnormality around the whole circumference. The surface is darker, irregular and may be bleeding. If possible the scope will be pushed gently past the tumour to check its dimensions. Sometimes the growth is of a size which prevents passage of the scope past it. The surgeon will pass a special pair of forceps through the sigmoidoscope to snip off a small piece of the lump (a biopsy) so that the pathologist can examine it, firstly to confirm the diagnosis and, secondly, to try to gauge the aggressiveness of the malignancy. Biopsy is painless: the patient is usually not aware that this is happening. Sometimes, instead of the usual rigid scope, the surgeon will use a longer, flexible fibreoptic sigmoidoscope at the routine out-patient visit. This has the advantage of reaching up into the descending colon, thus being able to examine directly and to biopsy a greater proportion of tumours.

Having completed these examinations the surgeon will often have a very clear idea of the problem. Further investigations will depend on what information is already to hand from the history and examination. For instance, if:

• *a tumour has been seen through sigmoidoscope*, the surgeon will probably arrange a barium enema X-ray (see below) to check the state of the rest of the bowel, as there is a 3 per cent chance there there is a second cancer present elsewhere. He or she is likely to tell the patient that a growth may be present, pending pathological confirmation, and that an operation is likely to be needed.

• *a tumour has not been seen but suspicions are strong, based on the findings*, the surgeon will arrange further investigation, either a barium enema X-ray or a total colonoscopy, to check the whole colon beyond the reach of the sigmoidoscope. Most probably further discussion will be reserved until the patient returns for a further out-patient visit after the investigations have been performed.

Barium enema X-ray (see Plate 1)

This investigation is performed either to look for a suspected cancer beyond the reach of the sigmoidoscope, or to check that there is not a further growth elsewhere in the bowel in a patient already found to have a rectal cancer.

Before the X-ray examination can be performed the bowel needs to be 'prepared'. This involves clearing it of faeces to make interpretation of the X-ray pictures more straightforward. Bowel preparation is usually performed by giving the patient a sachet of powder to take by mouth at home the day before the examination; this causes a period of frequent, loose bowel actions, after which the bowel is usually empty of faeces. Sometimes patients are given an enema (a fluid medication inserted into the rectum through a soft rubber tube) on arrival just to be sure that the bowel is empty.

Normally the bowel cannot be seen on X-ray pictures as the rays pass straight through it. The principle behind a barium enema X-ray is that by introducing a solution of barium sulphate into the bowel which shows up on the X-ray pictures, the anatomy becomes visible, so any abnormalities can be noted. Barium sulphate looks rather like, and has the consistency of, single cream. This is run into the rectum through a soft rubber tube; by tipping and turning the patient it is possible to get the barium to pass around the whole rectum and colon. By introducing some air as well, the inside surface of the bowel becomes coated with a very thin layer of the barium solution so that surface detail is shown more clearly. The whole examination usually takes around 30 minutes; it may be a little uncomfortable, mainly due to distension of the bowel with air, but it should not be painful. On X-raying the abdomen the bowel and the fine details of its lining show up very clearly. Any lumps or narrowings can be detected. Lumps as small as a few millimetres in diameter can be seen. After the examination, the patient is likely to pass barium from the bowel for a day or two, making the faeces white. The radiologist will not be able to give an immediate verdict on the examination, preferring to spend some time at the end of the session examining the pictures prior to writing a report for the surgeon.

Colonoscopy (see Plate 2)

This procedure involves the insertion of a long flexible instrument (colonoscope) to examine the surface lining of the whole colon and rectum; it has two advantages over barium enema X-ray examination, firstly it is more efficient at finding very small benign adenomas and cancers, and secondly it is possible to take biopsies and to remove adenomas if they are not too large.

Bowel preparation is needed, as for barium enema, so that the bowel wall can be examined easily. Usually the patient will be given an intravenous injection of Valium, or a similar drug, to sedate them. The patient is laid on the left side and the tip of the instrument is inserted through the anus. The colonoscopist is then able to guide the tip of the flexible scope by manipulating two controls on the eyepiece, all the while gently advancing the instrument into the bowel. In the average case the colonoscopist will be able to reach all the way to the caecum in about 15–20 minutes. If the scope comes up against a large tumour as it is inserted, it will not be possible to examine the whole bowel. The lining of the bowel will be examined most carefully as the scope is gently pulled back along the bowel. If a tumour is seen, a biopsy will be taken to confirm the diagnosis.

The patient rests in the department for a short while after the examination, after which they can go home, accompanied by a relative or friend, a necessary precaution if sedation has been used.

Scans

Other investigations are less frequently used. The most important are scans to examine the liver to look for secondary spread.

- **Ultrasound scan** (see Plate 3). This is the most frequently employed method, in which a beam of sound beyond the audible frequencies is directed into the body; tissues of different densities reflect the sound back differently. The returning sound is converted by computer into a 'map' on which the internal organs and abnormalities within them can be seen.
- **Computerized axial tomogram (CAT scan)** (see Plate 4). This procedure uses X-rays, and has the same aim as the ultrasound scan, but produces cross-sections of the body in greater detail; a CAT scan may sometimes be used to look at the rest of the abdomen and pelvis.
- **Radioimmune isotope scan** (see Plate 5). This involves the injection into the bloodstream of a harmlessly radioactive isotope in minute amounts, which is then taken up by various organs in the body. In recent years substances called monclonal antibodies, which are able to 'home in' on target tissues, especially cancers, have been

used experimentally to carry isotopes to the target issue. Using a 'gamma camera' the isotope can be detected to produce a map of isotope uptake in the abdominal organs. This method has allowed primary cancers to be shown up, but the technique is currently inferior to conventional barium enema and colonoscopic examination in this role; the technique may have a more useful place in the detection of recurrent tumours.

Pulling it all together

When all the necessary tests have been performed the patient will return to the out-patient department to see the surgeon again; at this stage information from the initial examination, and the results of X-rays, colonoscopy, scans, and any biopsies taken will be available. The surgeon should have a fair idea of the likely extent of the disease so that a full discussion with the patient can take place, including the treatment options.

The surgeon will discuss the results and his or her suggestions regarding treatment if a cancer has been confirmed. If the patient wishes, it is possible to have a relative or friend with them while seeing the surgeon for this consultation; this will provide support, and a second pair of ears to take in the information imparted by the doctor. For some patients it is easy to assimilate the information and to decide on the way forward, while for others the situation may be overwhelming and intimidating. The surgeon is at their disposal to try to clarify anything that remains obscure, but even after discussion the patient may wish to go away and talk to family, friends, and family doctor before going ahead with treatment. The patient should not feel pressurized into agreeing to a particular course of action; the surgeon should be the first to acknowledge the patient's need to go away and think it all through with the help of others before treatment is undertaken. If the patient wants to go ahead as arranged, the surgeon may be able to offer a date for admission, making the difficult period of waiting between the out-patient visit and treatment easier to cope with as there is at least a timetable agreed.

EMERGENCY HOSPITAL ADMISSION

Up to 30–40 per cent of all bowel cancer patients first visit the hospital as emergency cases, having developed one of the major complications, (bowel obstruction or perforation). Yet the majority of these patients will not have become suddenly ill from their bowel cancer. Around three-quarters will at an earlier stage have visited their family doctor with symptoms which turned out to have been due to the bowel condition. This highlights the difficulty sometimes in recognizing the serious nature of bowel symptoms which overlap with those produced by the much less serious and more common conditions.

Obstruction of the bowel causes the patient to develop severe cramping abdominal pain, accompanied by cessation of bowel action, distension of the abdomen and vomiting. Perforation of the bowel causes peritonitis, characterized by very severe abdominal pain which is constant and made worse by movement and by breathing. Here again there may be vomiting and distension of the abdomen. In both situations it is usually apparent to the patient and their relatives that he or she is very ill, leading to call out of the family doctor or even an emergency call summoning an ambulance.

The patient will be seen by one of the doctors in the Emergency Department who will begin the task of coming to a diagnosis and carrying out initial treatment. From a rapid appraisal of the symptoms and findings on examination, it should be possible to reach a diagnosis of bowel obstruction or perforation, though the precise cause can only be suspected at this stage. The doctor may decide that the patient is sufficiently ill to require resuscitation by means of an intravenous 'drip' before any further investigation is carried out. Some blood tests will be ordered, and X-rays of the abdomen and chest will be performed quickly. The X-ray films may show the tell-tale signs of distension of the bowel suggesting obstruction or peritonitis due to perforation. Gas which has escaped from the bowel may also be seen, clinching a diagnosis of perforation.

Having established that one of these diagnoses is likely, the doctor will call the surgeon, whose task it will be to decide on further treatment, almost certainly including an operation in the next 24 hours or so. Details of these decisions and of the treatment required in these circumstances will be found in Chapter 6 (see p. 112).

HEREDITARY DISEASES

In Chapter 3 (see p. 46), a group of hereditary conditions was mentioned in which some members of affected families are at increased risk of bowel cancer. The care of such families deserves special mention. One condition, familial adenomatous polyposis, has a rather characteristic clinical pattern, while the other family conditions are not always obvious if only a single member of the family is examined; in these cases the clinical picture may be no different from that seen in the non-familial forms of bowel cancer.

Familial adenomatous polyposis (FAP)

Before describing the first visit to hospital for those who may have this condition, it would be appropriate to describe its various features more fully than has occurred so far in the book. Familial adenomatous polyposis (FAP) is a dominantly inherited disease, which means that each of the offspring of an affected person stands a 50:50 chance of inheriting the condition. About one in 10 000–25 000 live births carry this abnormality. It is usually reported as causing about 1 per cent of all cases of colorectal cancer in Western countries, most of which can be prevented by efficient identification and preventive surgical treatment. FAP may produce abnormalities in the tissues in many parts of the body, as follows.

Large bowel adenomas　The most striking change is the appearance of adenomata of the large bowel mucosa; these are usually extremely numerous (100s or 1000s) and progression to adenocarcinoma in one or more is almost certain to occur by the fifth decade if preventive surgery is not carried out. Colorectal adenomas usually appear in the early teenage years.

Upper gastrointestinal (GI) adenomas　The majority of affected individuals develop adenomas elsewhere in the intestine, particularly in the duodenum, and less commonly in the stomach, bile duct or gall bladder (Fig. 3, p. 6). Fundic gland polyps, another sort of polyp with no cancer risk, may also occur in the stomach. Upper GI adenomas may become malignant.

Benign lesions of the skin, bones, and eyes　Most affected people will have a variable number of skin cysts, benign bone tumours, particularly of the jaw, and pigmented spots on the retina, at the back of the eye. None of these lesions carries any threat to life or health, but may serve as useful diagnostic markers in some cases.

Plates

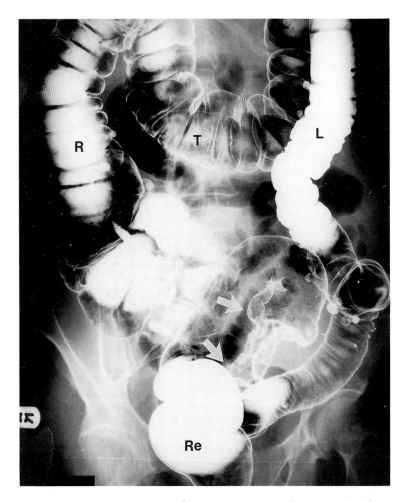

Plate 1. Barium enema X-ray, showing a cancer in the sigmoid colon.
This shows the picture obtained by a double-contrast barium enema, in
which a mixture of barium (white) and air (grey/black) has been injected
through the anus to show up the outline of the bowel (compare the
appearances with Fig. 3(b), p. 6). In the rather long sigmoid colon there is
a cancer (between the two arrows). At this point the bowel is narrowed and
irregular. The shape of the abnormal area gives rise to the term 'apple core
deformity', and is typical of a bowel cancer. (R: right colon; T: transverse
colon; L: left colon; Re: rectum).

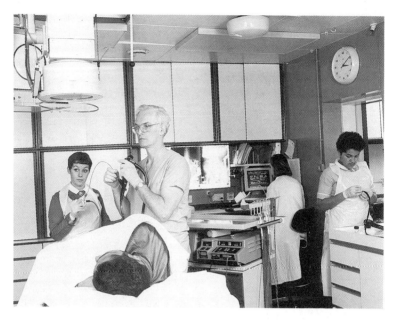

Plate 2. The colonoscopist at work. The colonoscopist works with a team of nurses particularly skilled in this type of work. The long, flexible instrument has been passed into the patient's bowel via the anus. Sometimes the colonoscopist examines the view by looking through the upper end of the instrument, like using a telescope. In this case a modern conoloscope is producing a high-definition television picture, which the doctor and nurse are looking at. A long, very thin biopsy forceps has been slid through a channel within the colonoscope; under direct vision, they can watch as they take a sample of tissue for pathological examination from deep within the bowel. The nurse on the right is cleaning a colonoscope after use.

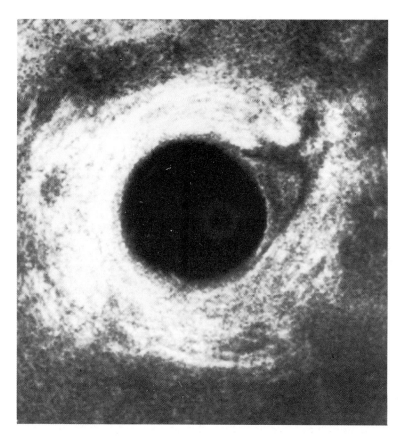

Plate 3. Ultrasound scan of the rectum. This scan is made by inserting a narrow probe into the rectum. It emits high-frequency sound which is reflected back to varying degrees by different tissues. A computer can then produce a cross-sectional picture. The dark area in the centre contains a water-filled balloon, with the probe at its centre. The general pattern of the tissues of the rectal wall and its surrounding structures is interrupted by the darker triangle, representing a cancer growing outwards through the rectal wall. Using this technique, it is possible to gauge the depth of spread of the cancer, and sometimes to get an idea of whether the nearby lymph glands are involved.

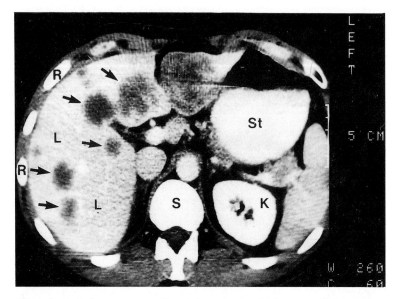

Plate 4. CAT (computerized axial tomographic) scan of the upper abdomen. This type of X-ray examination allows the radiologist to look at the patient in cross-section. This picture includes the rib cage (R), liver (L), the stomach (St), and the left kidney (K); a spinal vertebra (S) is seen in the lower part of the picture. The dark patches (arrowed) within the liver should not be there—these are most likely to be secondary cancers ('metastases') in a patient already known to have a primary cancer in the bowel. This diagnosis can be confirmed by taking samples of cells from one of the dark areas, using the scan to direct the collecting needle to the right spot under local anaesthesia.

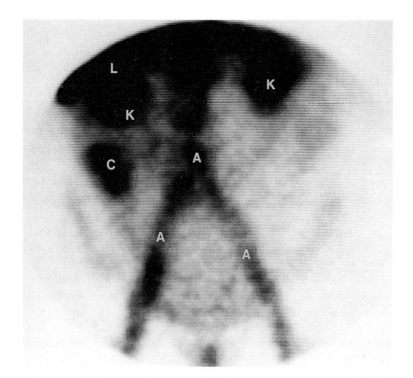

Plate 5. Radioimmune isotope scan. This uses an ingenious method for detecting a bowel cancer. A 'monoclonal antibody', a substance which is able to home in on a cancer, has been chemically bonded to a radioactive chemical, an 'isotope'. By this method a concentration of the isotope occurs in the cancer (C), which can be detected and recorded, as in this picture, using a 'gamma camera'. The chemical mixture can also be seen to highlight the large arteries in the abdomen (A), the kidneys (K), and the liver (L). One day it may become common practice to use monoclonal antibodies to carry poisons to tumours in order to destroy them.

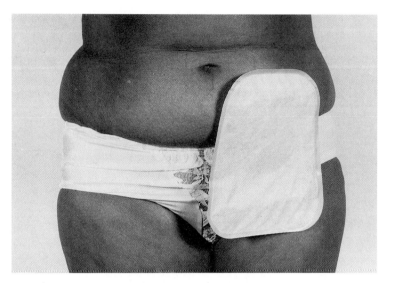

Plate 6. A colostomy appliance in position. This colostomy is in the most common site, the left iliac fossa. This is the position chosen when the rectum has been removed. The stoma is placed so that it can be dealt with easily by the patient, and lies above the usual position for her underwear. It is also sited away from the umbilicus (belly button) and the bony prominence of the pelvis to its left.

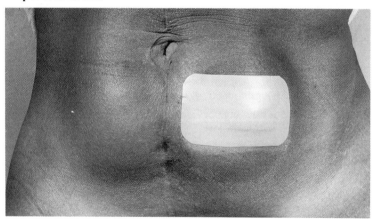

Plate 7. Colostomy dressing in a patient who irrigates. For those patients who irrigate their colostomy successfully (see page 149), a conventional colostomy bag is not needed. Instead, some people use a mini-bag, while others, such as this patient, simply apply an adhesive dressing after irrigation.

Desmoid tumours (including 'mesenteric fibromatosis') Fibrous
tumours, which may or may not cause symptoms, may grow in the
peritoneal cavity (particularly in the small bowel mesentery), abdominal
wall, or (less frequently) elsewhere in the body. Although they do not
metastasize, they may infiltrate locally, damaging bowel, mesenteric
blood vessels, ureters, etc., causing life-threatening complications.

Rarer malignancies Cancers of the adrenal and thyroid glands and of
the brain and liver have also been reported in FAP sufferers.

The first out-patient visit

What happens on the initial visit to the specialist for those with this
condition depends on the individual circumstances. Sometimes the
person will have no family history of this condition, which has arisen in
them due to a 'fresh mutation' (see below). For others the family history
of this condition will be well known to them, and they will be attending
to be examined to see if they have inherited the abnormality.

The fresh mutation As this condition is caused by a single abnormal
gene (millions of genes in each body cell carry all the details of our
inherited characteristics), it can arise spontaneously if by chance a person
develops a sudden change in their previously normal 'polyposis gene'. In
these circumstances none of their brothers, sisters, or parents would
develop this condition, but each of their children will have a 50:50
chance of inheriting FAP. Such a person may attend hospital having
noticed bleeding or change in bowel regularity. On examination the surgeon's suspicions will be roused by the multiple polyps seen in the
rectum on sigmoidoscopy, and perhaps the relatively young age of the
patient. If a barium enema or a colonoscopy reveals countless polyps, and
if pathological examination shows a sample polyp to be an adenoma, the
diagnosis is all but clinched. In some people in this situation cancer may
already have developed. A further check on the family history will reveal
no family history of bowel disease; to be sure that there is no other case in
their immediate family, any brothers, sisters, or parents may be advised
to attend for a check, requiring no more than a sigmoidoscopy. In the
absence of any signs of the condition in other family members, the
diagnosis of fresh mutational FAP is likely to be made, and the patient
advised to undergo surgery to diminish the cancer risk (see p. 115). The
patient will be advised that their offspring are at risk of inheriting FAP,

so at the appropriate time they will be offered examination to try to detect FAP at an early stage, should it develop.

The established affected family   Once a family has been shown to harbour the gene for FAP, it is of great importance that anyone at risk should be known to a hospital caring for other family members so that they can be advised about appropriate surveillance. As the first abnormalities in the bowel do not usually appear until the early teenage years, there is no need to examine at-risk children until they are around 14 years old.

When a child is brought along for their first visit they and their parents are naturally apprehensive, there being roughly a 50:50 chance that they will be found to have the condition. The doctor will ask a few simple questions about bowel function, though it is unlikely that any symptoms will have developed at this stage, even if polyps are present. Examination will include a search of the skin for the small cysts that may accompany the condition, and perhaps an examination of the eyes for small symptomless black spots that may occur on the retina in FAP. But the most important examination is a sigmoidoscopy, looking for the multiple bowel polyps which characterize the condition. If polyps are present, they will be biopsied to prove that they are adenomas, confirming the diagnosis. If no polyps are seen, the child will be brought back for re-examination the following year. As the years pass, if no polyps develop, the risk that they will appear diminishes, so that failure of polyps to appear by the age of 20 years reduces the risk of the ultimate development of FAP to around 3 per cent, or less than 1 in 30.

If a child is found to have developed the condition, a careful and detailed discussion with the child and the parents ensues. This is aimed at explaining the significance of the condition, though the parents are only too likely to be aware of this already. A decision needs to be made about treatment. By removing the bulk of the polyp-bearing bowel and keeping a close eye on what is left, the risk of cancer is greatly diminished. There are two operations used today, 'colectomy and ileorectal anastomosis' and 'restorative proctocolectomy', both of which aim to maintain normal bowel function via the rectum; the details of these will be discussed in Chapter 7 (see p. 118). Suffice at this stage to say that there is no need for undue haste in performing this surgery as the cancer risk in the teens is very low. The operation is usually advised for a time which will cause the minimum of disruption to the developing child, preferably during a summer holiday period, and in a year in which school examinations, or preparation for them, are not going to be disturbed too much by a spell in hospital followed by a period of recuperation. Following this treatment, patients return to a normal life, capable of all the activities of their friends at school or work.

Genetic counselling

The millions of genes in each cell are arranged in long strings called chromosomes. Recent research has located the polyposis gene on chromosome 5. By taking blood samples from several members of the family to track the inheritance of 'gene markers', which lie close to the polyposis gene, it is now possible in many cases to tell whether an individual family member is likely to be carrying the abnormal polyposis gene. This might be useful in several situations:

1. **The child at risk.** Parents might wish to know as early as possible whether their child is likely to become affected, rather than wait to see if polyps develop in the teenage years. This would either set the child's and their minds at rest if the abnormality is found not to be present, or perhaps take the uncertainty out of the situation and allow them all to get used to the idea at an early stage if the abnormal gene is confirmed.

2. **The apparently unaffected young person wishing to marry.** It is important to remember that only those who carry the gene can pass it on to their offspring. The young person who has not developed polyps (yet who might nevertheless carry the gene and develop polyps a little later than usual), having reached, say, the age of 20, might wish to be able to tell their intended spouse whether they are at risk of producing affected children. Although by this stage the risk has diminished, use of genetic probing might put the whole matter to a point almost beyond doubt.

3. **Pre-natal diagnosis.** Today it is possible to take a small sample from the tissue around the fetus in the uterus to check for genetic abnormalities; it should soon be possible to do this for an FAP-affected couple, so that they can be told whether the fetus is likely to be affected by FAP. If this test were performed early in pregnancy there might be the option to seek abortion if the fetus were likely to be affected. For those with a traumatic experience of the disease in their family, this facility might be an important comfort and safeguard while trying to share the normal joys of making a family.

All of these matters raise issues which require careful, sympathetic discussion. This is best achieved by a clinical geneticist, a doctor experienced in counselling on the problems of genetic diseases, and who will be in the best position to help those who wish to make use of the genetic probes as they become available.

Cancer family syndromes

Whereas FAP produces a very distinctive set of abnormalities in those affected, particularly the very large number of polyps in the bowel, the other inherited abnormalities which can give rise to bowel cancer do not; the individual member of an affected family will develop changes which are very much like those in people who contract cancer due to non-genetic causes. So picking out the affected family is not as easy as in FAP. So how are individuals and families to know that they should visit a doctor for genetic advice? Evidence suggests that the following factors raise the chances that a family might be harbouring a genetic abnormality which predisposes to bowel cancer.

1. Two or more first degree relatives (parents, brothers, sisters, children) have suffered from bowel cancer or one of the cancers which also occur in the Cancer Family Syndrome (particularly breast or ovarian cancer).
2. One family member has developed bowel cancer before the age of 45 years.

Members of families in which either of these patterns has occurred are best advised to see a clinical geneticist, who will take a very detailed family history looking for evidence of any of the cancers which may run in families. If the person has symptoms they will be referred to a surgeon for investigation; if they have no symptoms, the geneticist will try to assess their likely individual risk and suggest a programme of surveillance to try to prevent them from ever developing cancer. If they have a risk worse than one in ten of developing bowel cancer, the geneticist will probably advise colonoscopy at three or five yearly intervals to check for the presence of adenomas; if these are found they can be removed at the same sitting, thus preventing their possible progression to malignancy (see p. 80). For female members of cancer families, breast and ovarian screening may also be advised.

So far there are no genetic probe tests which can be used as in FAP to indicate whether an individual is carrying the abnormal gene; this would make the job of confirming family and individual risk much easier. However, it is highly likely that this powerful tool will be found at some stage in the fairly near future.

SUMMARY

Now we have looked at the various ways in which a patient with bowel cancer, or one of the associated conditions is likely to be cared for in the process of coming to a firm diagnosis. The time has now come to look at the various ways in which the condition can be dealt with; this will be explained in the next few chapters.

7
Surgery for bowel cancer

Although radiotherapy and chemotherapy may have a part to play in the treatment of some bowel cancer patients, the mainstay is still surgery. Operations for bowel cancer vary from relatively minor procedures, sometimes performed on an out-patient basis, to major operations taxing the technical expertise of the surgeon to its limits. Before looking at the way surgery may be used today in bowel cancer, we should start with a short account of the development of surgery in this disease.

HISTORY OF BOWEL CANCER SURGERY

Before the present century, bowel cancer was less common and treatment was rather rudimentary. In the late 1700s surgeons began making an 'artificial anus', or colostomy—an opening on the abdomen to allow faeces to escape—in some patients suffering from obstruction of the bowel due to cancer. This was then a highly dangerous exercise, aimed at relieving dire symptoms, with no prospect of curing the patient. In the early 1800s some surgeons resorted to pulling cancer tissue out through the anus to try to relieve patients afflicted by obstructing rectal cancers. By the late 1800s the lower part of the rectum was sometimes removed when it contained a cancer, leaving a gaping hole in the patient's bottom through which faeces would escape without control. The wound would usually have become infected and painful. The advanced stages of the disease must have been dreadful for patients and surgeons to conspire together in the undertaking of this procedure. Indeed, it seems that this sort of surgery was not universally well regarded—surgeon Henry Smith commented on it thus in 1870:

Some surgeons a few years since were in the habit of performing excision of the lower part of the rectum when affected by cancer, but this proceeding must be looked upon as both barbarous and unscientific, and is now happily exploded from the catalogue of surgical operations.

But the latter part of his statement was based in hope rather than fact, for it continued to be used. A colostomy, placed in the left lower part of the abdomen was added, which must have made it a little more tolerable for the recipients. Then, in 1908, Ernest Miles of the Gordon Hospital in London, described his operation for rectal cancer which still has a place in the 'catalogue of surgical operations' employed today. Miles' operation differed from the procedure described above in that the surgeon opened the abdomen, a considerable undertaking at that time, to remove a portion of the bowel and to make a colostomy. He then turned the patient on his or her side and completed the operation by working from below as described above, allowing the rectum and the cancer within it to be removed from below. The big difference between this and the earlier procedure was that it allowed the surgeon a good view of the cancer, so that he could attempt a radical (i.e. potentially curative) excision. Cure, said Miles, was possible for the first time; but at considerable cost. Forty per cent of Miles' patients died at, or soon after, the operation. It was to be another 30 years before general care of the surgical patient had reached a level at which many surgeons felt that the procedure was widely applicable.

Towards less severe operations

In the 1920s pathologists examining the surgical specimens removed from rectal cancer patients, gradually became aware of something that was to lead to an important change in surgery—towards less mutilating operations in which a colostomy could be avoided. They found that the lymphatic drainage of the rectum was almost exclusively *upwards*, away from the anus, so that the lower part of the rectum did not have to be removed as a routine in order to gain adequate clearance of the tumour. The bowel ends, therefore, could be rejoined and the patient could expect to have normal bowel function after surgery. The idea that rectal cancer could be cured without removing the whole rectum was regarded by many as dangerous heresy in the late '30s and '40s, but gradually it came to be seen as acceptable. The development of surgical techniques meant that more patients could undergo 'sphincter-saving surgery', i.e. operations in which anal sphincters (see p. 15), and hence continence, were preserved; today around 50–75 per cent of rectal cancer patients who are seen as candidates for attempts at cure can undergo surgery which leaves their sphincters intact.

The fibreoptic revolution

Another important step forward began outside medical practice and
science: this was the development in the '50s and '60s of fibreoptic
technology, whereby thousands of minute glass fibres could be held
together in a bundle, each transmitting faithfully along its length the
light which it picked up at its other end. Using this advance, long flexible
'endoscopes' were developed which could transmit a whole image, made
up of all the little spots of light transmitted from one end of the glass fibre
bundle to the other, no matter what twists and turns were imposed along
its length. This new family of instruments were sometimes known as
'fibre endoscopes', or 'fibrescopes', instruments which could be inserted
through any orifice in a patient—mouth, anus, urethra, etc.—to allow a
view of the inside. In the case of the large bowel the instrument was
called a colonoscope, which could be passed through the anus and around
the rectum and colon to allow a good view of the lining of the bowel.
Disease could be seen, including tumours, and biopsies taken using long
wire forceps. In some cases small tumours could actually be treated by
passing electrified cutting 'lassos' along the scope. This could be done on
the unanaesthetized patient without even admitting them to the wards.

SURGICAL MANAGEMENT TODAY

The surgeon treating bowel cancer patients today has a wide range of
techniques and tools available to deal with the many different situations
that may prevail. Patients may present with a gradual onset of symptoms
causing them at some stage to seek medical advice, which leads them to
the out-patient department. After complete investigation of symptoms
and establishment of the diagnosis, the patient may undergo 'elective'
surgery, i.e. the surgeon is able to 'elect' to operate at a time (usually
within a week or two) when the patient has been properly prepared for
surgery. Others present as an emergency, due to the sudden onset of a
major complication of the disease. Management in these two categories
differs substantially, so they will be discussed separately.

ELECTIVE SURGERY

Principles of cancer surgery

A radical cancer operation aims to remove the primary tumour, the
lymphatic tissue through which drains the body fluid released within the

tissues in and around the primary tumour, and a margin of normal tissue around the tumour and lymphatic tissue, sufficient to ensure the best chance that all tumour cells have been removed and therefore that the patient has been given the best chance of a cure. These principles were put forward by an American surgeon, William Halsted, at the end of the last century and Ernest Miles applied them to rectal cancer surgery soon afterwards.

In some cases the surgeon will find at operation that the tumour has spread so far that potentially curative radical surgery is not possible. In these circumstances the overriding aim is to do whatever is appropriate to keep the patient comfortable. Any such treatment is described as 'palliative'; surgery in this context will be discussed specifically in a later section.

Preparation for surgery

Before elective surgery can be carried out in a bowel cancer patient, they need to be admitted to hospital to prepare them for surgery. This will include checking on their general health (to be sure that they are fit for a general anaesthetic), preparing the bowel for surgery, and trying to ensure that they are clear as to what is planned, and mentally prepared for the experience to come.

General health check
The house surgeon (intern), usually the youngest member of the surgical team, has as one of his or her major tasks the routine, thorough checking of the general health of the patients admitted under their consultant. This will involve a very careful discussion of the immediate health problem and past illnesses, a full examination, and the ordering of appropriate investigations, such as blood tests, chest X-ray, electrocardiogram, etc., all of which is subsequently discussed with the more senior members of the surgical team. The day before surgery it is likely that the anaesthetist will come along to look at the information gleaned by the house surgeon (intern) and to examine the patient again.

Bowel preparation
In order to make bowel surgery as safe as possible it is necessary to cleanse the bowel of faecal material. This decreases the risk of spillage of faeces during surgery and of disruption of any stitches in the bowel wall during the postoperative period. There are several methods available for bowel preparation:

- **Laxatives and wash-outs.** In this method the patient takes one or two doses of a strong laxative 24–36 hours before operation, followed by a simple enema to make sure the rectum is empty on the morning of the operation.
- **Irrigation.** This technique involves the passage of a small plastic tube via the nostril into the stomach (nasogastric tube), followed by the drip feed of several litres of salt solution. This washes the bowel through very thoroughly; the patient passes the large volumes of saline together with all faecal matter over a variable period of hours. Some patients find this method rather taxing, but it certainly works very well.
- **Mannitol.** Mannitol is a type of sugar. When a solution of this substance is either drunk or instilled into the stomach via a tube it acts as a strong laxative, causing the passage of very fluid motions until the bowel is free of faeces.

To some extent all methods of bowel preparation produce discomfort for the patient; stimulation of the bowel may cause cramps and a bloated feeling. But such preparation is necessary to make the operation as clean, and therefore as safe, as possible.

Preventing blood clots

As with all major surgery there is a risk of blood clots forming in the veins in the legs. There is a small but definite risk that these may break free and travel in the blood stream to the lungs, where they can, if large enough, block the circulation causing severe acute illness or even death. In order to minimize this risk many surgeons prescribe regular small doses of heparin, a drug which makes the blood less able to clot. This is given by injection under the skin, usually of the abdomen or thigh. Another way to decrease the risk of clotting is the use of elasticated stockings which speed up the flow of blood in the leg veins.

Meeting the stoma care nurse

Many hospitals have a specialist nurse on the staff, the **stoma care nurse**, whose only task is to help in the care of patients preparing for, or learning to live with, a colostomy or ileostomy. If the forthcoming operation is likely to require a stoma, this nurse will visit before operation. His or her tasks at this stage are to help to familiarize the patient with this aspect of the operation and to choose the best site for the opening, and to mark it carefully. He or she will show the patient the sort of appliance to be used, and may stick it onto the skin so that the patient has some idea how it will feel. If it seems useful in any particular case, the stoma care nurse will be able to arrange for someone who already has a similar stoma to make a visit, to offer assurance and first hand experience to the apprehensive patient. This nurse is an invaluable ally to the stoma patient; there will be more details on stoma care in chapter 9 (see p. 146).

The physiotherapist

Inactivity and difficulty in movement are usual in the immediate post-operative period, and predispose to chest infections, blood clots, etc. Physiotherapy helps the recovering patient to resume activity as comfortably and as early as possible, thus decreasing the risk of such complications. The physiotherapist, who is skilled in teaching and supervising these activities, will usually make a visit before operation to explain what is to come, and to begin teaching some simple breathing and movement exercises.

Discussion of surgery

An important part of the preoperative preparation of the patient is the discussion with the surgeon of the procedure planned, and its likely outcome. This is the time for the patient to make sure that he or she gets answers to any remaining questions about the disease and its treatment. One thing the surgeon may be unable to do at this stage is to give a strong indication of the chance of cure. Examination and investigations may have shown already that widespread incurable disease is present, but often the surgeon will not find this out until the operation is under way. Furthermore, the pathologist will be able to provide additional information on the prospects for cure after examination of the operative specimen. The surgeon should remind the patient of the principles of the operation and of the degree of likelihood of a colostomy, and its possible siting. The surgeon is also likely to warn the patient of any particular complications that might occur. Hopefully, this part of the discussion will be conducted with delicacy and skill, for the patient already has enough frightening things to think about without the burden being increased unnecessarily. The surgeon is likely to emphasize the relatively small risk of most of these complications, while pointing out any which seems more important or relevant for this individual patient. So, while remembering that the risks of complications are generally fairly low, it is worth looking at what the surgeon may discuss in a little detail.

Possible complications

These days, elective bowel cancer surgery carries a smaller risk of post-operative complications than used to be the case. The possible problems can be divided into general complications that can occur after any major operation, and special ones related directly to bowel surgery.

General complications

All major abdominal surgery carries a risk of problems related to the circulation ('heart attack', stroke), the lungs (chest infection, blood clot), the urinary system (infection or difficulty with emptying the bladder), and the operation wound (infection or 'dehiscence'—complete separation of the wound edges). These are kept to a minimum by careful preoperative assessment for risk factors, and active attempts to prevent them by such measures as physiotherapy. If the patient is a smoker, they are at increased risk of chest complications. Therefore, he or she will be encouraged to stop, as even a short break before operation helps the lungs and airways to recover to some extent, making them more resistant to infection. Obesity is another important risk factor for all the complications listed above; although encouragement to lose weight may be appropriate before surgery for less urgent conditions, it is not usually possible in the bowel cancer patient.

Special complications

Anastomotic leakage When two lengths of bowel are joined together after removal of an intervening segment containing a cancer, the join is called an anastomosis; a minor degree of leakage from this join is fairly common and non-threatening but in a few cases is potentially very dangerous. Most anastomoses heal uneventfully despite faeces passing through the operated bowel within a few days of operation. Generally, if the surgeon feels that a particular anastomosis is at significant risk of leaking, he or she will make a temporary, 'defunctioning' colostomy 'upstream' to rest the sutured bowel while it heals. Sometimes, however, an anastomosis which did not seem to be at risk of leaking, and was therefore not protected by defunctioning colostomy will, nevertheless, spring a leak. This is probably due to infection around the site of the join, aggravated perhaps by the presence of a small collection of fluid or blood clot. If the surgeon has inadvertently damaged the blood supply to the joined bowel ends, this may also lead to an anastomotic leak. An un-noticed technical problem with the joining of the bowel ends may also

lead to leakage. A leak can manifest itself in various ways; most frequently it is small and produces no discomfort for the patient. A minor
leak may only be apparent because the surgeon has ordered a routine
X-ray around 7–10 days postoperatively to check on the integrity of the
anastomosis; it may produce no symptoms at all. Nothing needs to be
done about such a leak; it heals up spontaneously. On other occasions
the patient may develop a temperature, perhaps some abdominal discomfort and the bowel may become sluggish, causing nausea, decreased
bowel movements and distension of the abdomen. The body's defences
usually deal with this sort of leak by wrapping protective tissue around
the affected area, preventing spreading infection. In rare instances the
situation is more serious, with leakage of faeces throughout the abdominal cavity or out to the surface, perhaps through the surgical wound, or
both. This serious complication will frequently require further surgery to
clean the abdominal cavity and to make the bowel safe, usually by
making a temporary colostomy to prevent further uncontrolled leakage.

Nerve damage   As mentioned in the later operative section (see p. 105),
it may be necessary sometimes to remove some nerves which run on the
walls of the pelvis in order to gain adequate clearance in removing a
rectal cancer. If this has occurred it is likely to cause one or two particular
problems. First, the patient may not be able to pass urine spontaneously
because the bladder muscle does not receive the appropriate message to
contract and squeeze out the urine, while the sphincter muscle, which
normally relaxes to allow the bladder to empty, may not be able to
function properly. This difficulty requires placement of a tube in the
bladder (a catheter); this will be via the urethra initially, though if it
appears that it will be needed for a while it may be inserted through the
front of the lowest part of the abdomen as this is more comfortable and
convenient. The bladder sometimes recovers spontaneously, perhaps
with the help of medication, though on other occasions a specialist in
urinary problems (a urologist) may need to be consulted; he or she will
probably test bladder function and then either prescribe medication to
encourage bladder emptying or perform a small operation to restore
urinary flow.

The other way in which nerve damage can manifest itself is impotence
and/or sterility in the male; it seems that women do not usually develop
an equivalent sexual failure. 'Impotence' refers to failure of erection,
while 'sterility' indicates failure of ejaculation. The risk of sexual nerve
damage varies with the operation—total removal of the rectum is more

likely to cause such damage than partial removal—the reason for this difference is that some of the tissues containing the nerves are left undisturbed in the lesser procedure. The proportion of patients suffering this problem after surgery varies in reports from different surgeons. It is important when looking at reports of sexual problems after surgery to note the extent of sexual activity *before* operation. This may explain reports of 100 per cent sexual dysfunction when all age groups are considered, compared to around 40 per cent in patients under 50 years of age; it has been suggested that the higher figure in the 'all comers' group may reflect a higher proportion with preoperative impotence, thus inflating the apparent deleterious effect of surgery. Other factors which may contribute to postoperative sexual problems include psychological problems. In this case there may be some improvement with time, but if there has been actual damage to nerves, recovery is unlikely. There are specialist urological centres which are able to offer some help in the treatment of impotence after pelvic surgery.

Summary
In summary, the patient will spend a rather hectic couple of days in hospital prior to surgery, undergoing preparation for, and explanation of, what is to come. At the end of this phase they should have met all those who will be involved in their care, will have been rendered as fit as possible for surgery, and will have had adequate explanation of the disease, its treatment and the train of events unfolding around them.

What happens on operation day?

After a night when sleep will probably have been difficult, though perhaps made easier with sleeping tablets, the day of operation arrives. About one hour prior to the time of the operation, the nurses on the ward will give the patient some preoperative medication—the 'pre-med'. This is usually in the form of an injection in the buttock or leg, aimed at rendering the patient sleepy and at ease, and drying up the secretions in the mouth and air passages, making the anaesthetic safer. At the appropriate time, the trip to the anaesthetic room will be made on a trolley brought to the ward by the theatre staff.

The anaesthetic room
Here the nurse who has accompanied the patient from the ward will carry out the very important task of confirming formally the patient's

identity to the theatre staff. The anaesthetist will then gently put the patient off to sleep with an injection in the back of the hand; the injection also contains a substance which completely paralyses all the muscles in the body. This makes it possible for the anaesthetist to take over the work of breathing using a machine which pumps exactly the right amount of oxygen, together with anaesthetic agents, into the lungs using a 'ventilator' and a tube placed in the main airway (an 'endotracheal tube'). Paralysis also makes it much easier for the surgeon to operate inside the abdomen. Having settled the patient into peaceful sleep, the anaesthetist will insert a 'drip' in a vein in the arm to allow fluids to be given during the operation, and a urinary catheter will be placed in the bladder to check on urine production. Keeping the bladder empty also makes it easier for the surgeon, especially if the rectum is the site of the tumour, as a full bladder obscures the view.

When all the preparations have been made, the patient is taken into the operating theatre and placed on the operating table ready for the surgeon to start the procedure.

The operation

The precise operation selected for the treatment of a bowel cancer will depend mainly on the site of the tumour, but whatever operation is to be carried out it has three main elements:

● the initial inspection of the bowel and other organs to assess the extent of the spread of the disease;
● removal of the primary tumour, and;
● either the rejoining (anastomosis) of the divided bowel or the formation of a colostomy.

These three elements will be dealt with separately.

Initial inspection

The abdomen is opened via an incision usually made vertically down the middle; sometimes it stretches from the lower end of the breast bone to the lower end of the abdomen, at the level of the pubic bone; usually, however, it is shorter than this, centred below or above the umbilicus ('belly button'), depending on the site of the primary tumour. The surgeon will then look at the expected site of the primary tumour to confirm the position and to check whether it has spread through the bowel wall. If it has spread through, it may have come to involve adjacent organs such as surrounding loops of bowel, the bladder, vagina, abdominal wall, etc. A check will also be made for distant spread, i.e. involvement of tissues not in direct continuity with the primary tumour; the two most likely sites for these 'secondary' tumours, or 'metastases', are the lining of the abdominal cavity (the peritoneum) and the liver. Peritoneal metastases usually consist of small whitish lumps a few millimetres in diameter; liver metastases appear as lumps of variable size within the liver substance. If they are deep within the liver, the surgeon may not be able to feel them, while those closer to the surface may be visible or palpable (i.e. they can be felt by the surgeon gently squeezing the liver).

Having carefully examined the abdominal contents the surgeon is now in a position to decide what can be done to help the patient. If there are peritoneal deposits or widespread liver involvement, the surgeon must come to the inevitable conclusion that curative treatment is impossible. Removal of the primary tumour is still likely to be worthwhile as the tumour will probably cause troublesome symptoms during the patient's remaining life if not removed. Before proceeding to remove the tumour the surgeon will take samples of tissue to confirm any distant spread that has been seen, as on rare occasions the surgeon will receive a surprise when the pathologist is able to say that the tissue thought to be spreading cancer is something quite benign and separate from the bowel cancer. Because of this slight possibility the surgeon would rarely contemplate telling the patient that they have advanced, incurable disease without pathological confirmation.

Getting the cancer out

This is the next step in the operation. As explained above, removal of the primary tumour includes taking away the lymphatic drainage of the tumour and a margin of normal tissue. If the tumour has invaded surrounding structures directly, the surgeon is faced with the decision as to whether it is possible to remove the whole growth together with any involved organs. Although such advanced cancers have a worse outlook, some can be cured, so it is none the less worth the attempt to remove them despite the possible consequences, such as the need to construct an artificial bladder.

This part of the operation differs, depending on the site of the cancer.

Colon cancer

Tumours of the colon are removed using operations referred to as 'colectomy' (Figs 9 and 10). A tumour involving the right or left side of

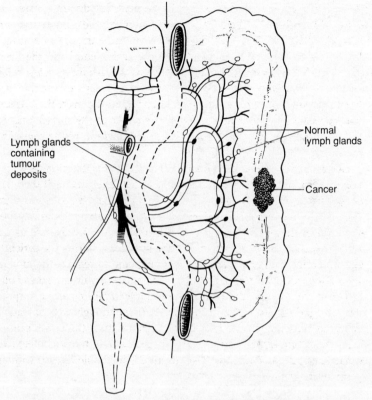

Fig. 9. Extent of operation to remove a cancer of the left colon. The arrows and the dotted lines indicate the line along which the surgeon cuts away the segment of bowel, and the lymph glands and arteries connected with it. Such wide removal is necessary to try to clear away any lymph glands that might contain tumour. (For simplicity the veins have not been shown.)

the colon will be removed by a procedure in which the affected half of the colon is taken (right or left hemi ('half') colectomy). Transverse colon cancer is removed by transverse colectomy and sigmoid colon cancer by sigmoid colectomy. The length of bowel removed is determined by the need to remove the lymph nodes draining the primary tumour. As these are situated along the main arteries supplying the region, the precise area to be removed is dictated by the routes of these vessels. In any colonic cancer operation ('resection') the surgeon begins by freeing the segment of bowel to be removed from the structures to which it is normally

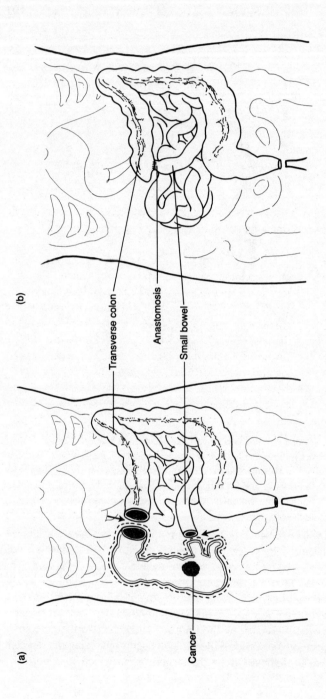

Fig. 10. Right hemicolectomy. (a) Extent of resection. As in Fig. 9, a wide clearance is necessary to maximize the chance of cure. (b) After anastomosis (rejoining of the bowel ends). The cut end of the small bowel has been stitched to the cut end of the transverse colon. The bowel resumes its normal function rapidly after such surgery.

attached: this allows the bowel to be lifted forwards into a more accessible position. The mesentery, the sheet of tissue containing the blood vessels supplying and draining the bowel segment, is normally adherent to the back of the abdominal cavity. Having mobilized the bowel, the surgeon can separate its mesentery quite easily; during this step he or she has to be careful not to damage other nearby structures. Having freed the mesentery, the main arteries and veins of the mobilized bowel, which lie within the mesentery, can be tied where they arise from, or drain into, the superior and inferior mesenteric arteries and veins.

The bowel segment to be removed is now free from all attachments except the bowel itself 'upstream' and 'downstream'. The surgeon has only to divide the bowel carefully at the chosen points, and the segment containing the tumour is free and ready to go to the pathologist.

Rectal cancer

It is a common misconception that treatment of rectal cancers requires that the patient be left with 'a bag'. Although this was once true, today at least 50 per cent of rectal cancer patients can be operated on without the need for a permanent colostomy. In these cases the diseased segment is removed and the bowel ends are rejoined, leaving the patient able to pass bowel motions in the normal way. If the whole rectum must be removed, the operation is called an 'abdomino-perineal excision', indicating that the rectum is removed by two surgical teams working from different directions, via the abdomen and the perineum (the area between the buttocks and the legs, which includes the anus). The procedure in which the diseased area is removed and the bowel ends joined can be used for most tumours in the upper half of the rectum and many in the lower half; this type of operation is known as 'anterior resection', or 'sphincter saving resection'.

Abdomino-perineal excision   This was the operation first described in 1908 by Ernest Miles. It consists of the radical removal of the whole rectum and anal canal and the formation of a colostomy in the left lower part of the abdominal wall (Fig. 11).

The positioning of the patient for this procedure is very important. Having placed the patient flat on his or her back on the operating table, the legs are supported while that part of the table on which they would otherwise lie is removed. A special set of 'stirrups' is attached to the lower end of the table, allowing the patient's legs to be supported in a position which, by angling them upwards and apart, allows a second

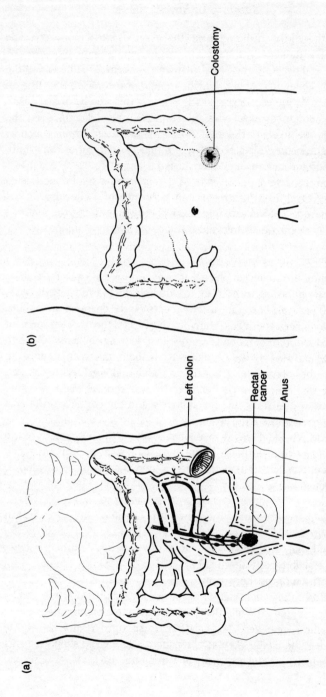

Fig. 11. Abdomino-perineal excision of the rectum. (a) Extent of resection. In this operation the whole rectum, anus, and part of the colon are removed, with the inferior mesenteric artery and its associated lymph glands. (b) Final result. The cut end of the colon is brought to the surface to form a colostomy.

surgeon to operate on the perineum. When the second surgeon is satisfied that the patient has been positioned satisfactorily, he or she places a
stitch around the anus to close it completely; this prevents seepage of any
residual faecal matter (which would contaminate the operative field) from
the rectum during the operation.

The operation begins with the freeing, or 'mobilization', of the upper
part of the rectum and the lower part of the sigmoid colon via a long
abdominal incision. The major artery and vein supplying the rectum
from above are cut across close to the aorta. The bowel is cut across in
the lower part of the sigmoid colon, leaving the lymphatic drainage of the
rectum attached to the segment of bowel to be removed. Great care is
taken to preserve the nerves supplying the bladder and organs of sexual
function as they pass downwards into the pelvis behind the rectum (see
Chapter 1, p. 16). Preservation is usually possible so long as the tumour
is not invading out of the back of the rectum to involve the tissues which
contain these nerves. The operation then proceeds downwards into the
pelvis, aiming to remove all of the tissues to the sides of and behind the
rectum. The vagina in the female or the bladder and seminal vesicles
(small organs which produce some of the constituents of semen) in the
male, must be separated from the front of the rectum. The dissection is
carried deeply into the pelvis, to the level of the upper surface of the
muscular sheet known as the pelvic floor, which stretches across the
depths of the pelvis.

Meanwhile a senior surgical assistant begins to operate via the perineum. A circumferential incision is made a few centimetres around the
anus; this is deepened so that soon the lower surface of the pelvic floor is
reached. The two surgeons operating from opposite ends of the pelvis are
now separated only by this thin sheet of muscle; at this stage the perineal
operator divides this muscle circumferentially around the rectum, allowing the latter to be removed through the perineal wound.

All that remains is for the surgeons to close the large cavity left in the
pelvis, to close the abdominal wall and to make a colostomy (this will be
discussed in more detail later, see p. 119). A drainage tube is usually
placed in the pelvis to remove any discharge of blood that might collect,
as this would increase the risk of infection.

Anterior resection This is the name given to the operation in which
the surgeon removes the segment of bowel containing the tumour
together with its lymphatic drainage, but leaves the lowest part of the
rectum and anal canal in place (Fig. 12). The surgeon is then able to join

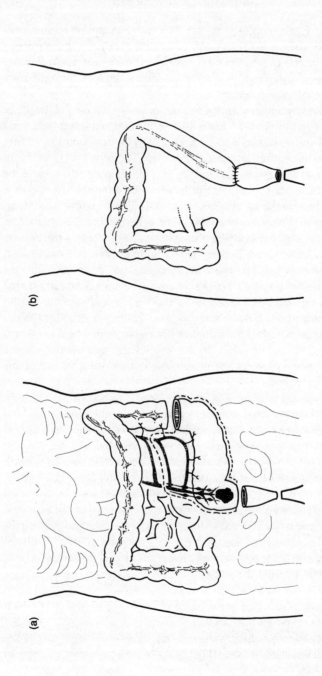

Fig. 12. Anterior resection of the rectum. (a) Extent of resection. This is the procedure if the rectal cancer can be removed safely without taking the lowest part of the rectum and anus. (b) After anastomosis. The cut end of the colon is joined to the remaining 'stump' of rectum. This is sometimes a very difficult procedure.

the healthy bowel ends together so that the patient will be able to pass motions normally again afterwards.

The early part of the operation—rectal mobilization—is the same as that used in abdomino-perineal excision. The surgeon needs to free the rectum from the surrounding tissues to a level several centimetres below the level of the tumour. As explained earlier, the lymphatic drainage of the tumour passes upwards towards the lymph glands around the aorta so that the surgeon is able to remove a minimum of tissue below the tumour and yet still be confident that the cancer has been removed safely. In order to cut across the bowel, the tissue carrying its blood vessels, which lies behind the rectum, has to be dissected, the blood vessels tied and the block of tissue cut through, leaving the rectum alone to be divided. When the rectum has been stripped like this, a clamp is placed across the bowel and a nurse passes a tube through the anus into the lower part of the rectum and washes it out with a solution which cleans out any remaining faecal matter and also, very importantly, kills any cancer cells that may be floating free within the bowel. This step makes joining the bowel ends together cleaner and safer, at the same time minimizing the risk of recurrence of the tumour due to growth of any residual cancer cells which might 'seed' on the cut bowel ends.

En bloc *removal of advanced tumours*   During initial assessment the surgeon will have discovered whether the tumour has invaded surrounding organs and, if so, whether the operation can be extended to remove all involved tissue. Any structure within the abdomen can be invaded directly by a spreading bowel cancer. The most commonly involved structures are the vagina, uterus, bladder, or small bowel. In these circumstances the patient may still be cured by appropriate extension of the operation. The back of the vagina, the whole uterus, part or all of the bladder, or a length of small bowel (or sometimes several of these structures together) can be removed '*en bloc*' (i.e. in the same single block of tissue) with the affected bowel. If part of the small bowel or bladder are removed, the organ has to be repaired. This is usually simply a matter of joining the bowel ends or closing the bladder, but if the whole bladder has been taken away the patient will need an alternative way of passing urine. This involves the construction of an 'ileal conduit'—an artificial bladder made from a length of small bowel. The cut ends of the ureters, which carry urine down from the kidneys, are sutured to one end of the ileal conduit while the other end is brought to the surface of the abdomen where a stoma (urostomy) is fashioned, so that urine can drain freely into a plastic bag appliance.

Making good after removing the tumour—anastomosis or stoma

Having removed the tumour using one of the major procedures described above, the surgeon is then faced with the task of restoring the patient's anatomy as closely as possible to normal (Figs. 10 and 12). If a segment of colon or rectum has been removed, by joining the ends together, the function of the bowel can be returned to normal; if, however, the rectum and anus have been removed, a colostomy is necessary to allow the bowel to empty (Fig. 11).

The technical term for joining the bowel ends together is 'anastomosis'. This is a fundamental part of many operations within the abdomen, whether for cancer of the bowel or stomach, or for benign conditions of any part of the intestine. The surgeon has to join the ends in a way which will allow the bowel contents to pass freely and safely along the bowel without leakage from the join. Surgeons vary in the way they do this. There are many different stitching materials ('sutures') available and lots of ways of using them to achieve a satisfactory result. In general, surgeons join the bowel ends either by placing a single ring of sutures around the join or by adding a second ring of sutures to bury the first. This is usually a very straightforward routine, but if the anastomosis is performed in the depths of the pelvis, especially in a fat person or in a male with a small pelvis, then the task can be one of the most difficult faced by a surgeon—it is rather like trying to perform this delicate task in the depths of a vase, often with poor lighting and using rather cumbersome, long instruments to hold the bowel ends and to insert the sutures. If at the end of this part of the operation the surgeon is unhappy about the quality of the anastomosis, he or she has the option of making a temporary stoma 'upstream' to divert faeces into a bag, so that the bowel content is temporarily prevented from flowing through the newly repaired bowel; the stoma can be closed a couple of months later when the anastomosis has been allowed to heal soundly.

Sometimes it is simply impossible to make the anastomosis at all using the conventional suture technique through the abdomen. Over the past 20 years, methods have been developed which allow an anastomosis to be constructed even under these difficult circumstances. First came the technique known as coloanal anastomosis in which the bowel ends are joined via the anus. By this method the whole of the lower rectum can be removed and still the ends can be joined—in fact the lower part *must* have been completely removed for this technique to be used. With the surgeon seated facing the perineum (the patient's legs held apart on stirrups), the surgeon's assistant delivers the upper cut end of the bowel down through the pelvis to the anus. The surgeon then places sutures between the bowel end and the anal canal. When this technique is used, the patient should always have a temporary stoma to protect the anastomosis while it heals. This method is followed by a tendency to frequent, rather loose stools in around 25 per cent of cases, though this usually settles as time passes. The other method which allows anastomosis under difficult circumstances entails the use of a stapling instrument. First developed by Russian surgeons many years ago, the method has become very popular in Western countries, where the details of the technique and design of the instruments have been advanced. Essentially the method allows the surgeon to attach the two cut ends of the bowel to the instrument, which looks rather like a gun, after it has been inserted through the anus (Fig. 13). On 'firing' the gun, two concentric rows of staples are automatically released which produce a secure anastomosis between the bowel ends. The steel staples may stay in place for ever— they cause no problems for the patient—or they may be shed silently into the faeces passing through the bowel months or years after their task of holding the bowel ends together during healing has been done. This technique has proved so successful that many surgeons use it for all rectal anastomoses. It is usual for low stapled anastomoses to be protected with a temporary stoma while the healing process of proceeding.

Surgery for liver metastases

As mentioned earlier, the surgeon may have discovered during pre-operative investigation, or during initial inspection at the beginning of the operation to remove the bowel tumour, that the liver is involved. Although this is generally a sign that cure is not possible, under some circumstances liver metastases can be dealt with surgically, giving the patient some chance of survival. Several recent studies have suggested that if there are only a few liver metastases (probably four or less) and they are confined to a single area of the liver, it may be possible to remove the affected area, with about a 30 per cent chance of cure. There is some argument amongst surgeons about whether this relatively favourable group might survive for several years anyway, without operation, but it is likely that at least some patients are cured by attempts to remove limited liver metastases.

It is usual, if the surgeon feels that a patient's liver metastases are potentially removable, to do this at a second operation, once the patient has recovered successfully from the first procedure to remove the primary

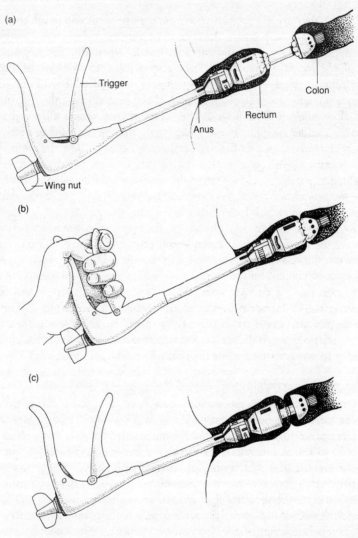

Fig. 13. Making an anastomosis using a 'staple gun'. (a) The staple gun is inserted through the anus and the two bowel ends are tied to the instrument. (b) The bowel ends are brought together using the 'wing nut' on the handle of the gun, and the gun is fired by squeezing the large 'trigger'. This releases many minute metal staples which join the bowel ends while at the same time a circular knife cuts out the disc of bowel tissue within the ring of staples, which allows; (c) release of the gun prior to its removal from anus. This leaves the bowel ends securely joined together.

bowel tumour. This will allow further investigation, in particular a CAT scan and X-rays of the layout of the arteries within the liver: these investigations help to confirm the limited nature of the metastases. Liver resection is a major undertaking. Depending on which part of the liver is to be removed, a large incision is made across the upper abdomen, often extending into the lower right side of the chest, to provide adequate access to the liver. Postoperatively the patient will spend some time in the intensive care unit while they begin to recover from this major operation.

Non-radical surgery

Occasionally a cancer is small enough to be treated by a 'non-radical' operation, i.e. one which removes only the primary tumour, leaving the lymphatic drainage field alone. This may be done by:

● local excision, or
● colonoscopic excision.

Local excision If the surgeon finds that the patient has a small cancer (up to 3–4 cm across) in the lower rectum, which does not appear to have invaded through the full thickness of the bowel wall, and if the out-patient biopsy indicates that the tumour is not of the most aggressive type, then he or she may be able to offer the patient this small operation instead of one of the much larger operations described above.

Local excision is performed with the patient anaesthetized and placed in the 'lithotomy' position (on their back with the legs held fully flexed in stirrups) or in the 'jack-knife' position (on their front with the table and the legs bent downwards in an upside down V shape allowing access to the anus). These positions allow tumours on the back and front walls of the rectum respectively, to be approached most easily. The surgeon can then expose the tumour by placing an instrument in the anus to hold it and the walls of the lower rectum widely open. After injecting adrenalin solution beneath the tumour to minimize bleeding, he or she cuts out a disc of bowel wall containing the tumour and a one centimetre cuff of normal tissue from around the cancer. The hole produced can then be sutured. The specimen is sent to the pathologist and the patient returns to the ward. A few days later, having fully assessed the specimen, the pathologist is able to tell the surgeon whether or not the tumour is at a sufficiently early stage and has been sufficiently well removed for the patient to be reassured that all is likely to be well. If, however, the pathologist has not been able to report favourably, the surgeon must visit the patient and suggest a conventional radical operation to ensure the best chance of cure.

Unfortunately only around 5 per cent of rectal cancers are at a sufficiently early stage when found, and located in a sufficiently accessible position, for local excision to be feasible.

Colonoscopic excision   The colonoscope, described earlier (see p. 80) in its role as a diagnostic tool, is also an extremely useful device for treating some small bowel cancers. When the tumour is on a stalk of normal tissue growing from the bowel wall, the colonoscope can be used to locate it and to 'lasso' it with a wire loop which can be tightened and through which an electric current can be passed to cut the cancer away. Colonoscopic removal is a straightforward procedure from the patient's point of view, carried out under mild sedation and with no need for a long stay in hospital afterwards. Of course, this method can only be used for this particularly favourable, and rather uncommon, type of early cancer. The method also allows the removal of benign adenomas, which might sometimes otherwise develop into cancers. Before the colonoscope was invented, open abdominal surgery was necessary to treat these conditions.

EMERGENCY SURGERY

It is a sad fact that 20–30 per cent of patients with bowel cancer consult a doctor for the first time having developed one of the complications of the disease. Of this group three-quarters arrive with acute obstruction of the colon while in the rest, the cancer has perforated, allowing bowel contents to escape, causing peritonitis. Both situations are potentially life-threatening, requiring a different approach to treatment than that employed following a more straightforward presentation.

Resuscitation and preparation for surgery

The obstructed bowel becomes loaded with large volumes of fluid, all of which has reached the bowel ultimately from the bloodstream, the digestive organs having made the digestive juices from the blood passing through them. This has the effect of reducing the blood volume, making the patient's general state rather poor as the heart works harder and harder to pump around the diminished volume of blood in order to supply food and oxygen to all the body's vital organs. The patient with peritonitis may go into a state of shock due to the inflammation in the abdomen. Both situations demand rapid assessment and treatment with intravenous fluid given through a drip in the arm. Patients are often unfit due to other health problems and these will need sorting out, with emergency treatment of these conditions as well, to make the impending surgery safer.

Aims of emergency surgery

The immediate aim of surgery in the emergency case is to save the patient's life; other considerations, including cure of the cancer, take second place for the moment. As with elective surgery, the emergency procedure can be thought of in three phases, initial assessment, dealing with the disease, and considering whether to perform an anastomosis or make a stoma.

Opening the abdomen and initial assessment

If the bowel is obstructed, special care is required when opening the abdomen as the tensely distended bowel can burst either due to damage by the scalpel or spontaneously when the support afforded to it by the surrounding abdominal wall is removed. If the bowel has perforated prior to operation, the surgeon's first task is to clean out the faeces that has leaked from the bowel. Much of the leaked material is fluid and can be removed with a suction device; when most of it has been cleared the surgeon will try to prevent further leakage by placing a gentle clamp across the bowel above the level of the leak. The remaining faecal material can then be washed out using several litres of warm saline solution.

The next step is to examine the cancer, checking the state of the primary tumour and looking for signs of spread elsewhere in the abdomen. Having done this, the surgeon must decide whether to remove the cancer at this operation or to do the minimum to sort out the emergency, and leave tackling the cancer for another day when the patient has recovered somewhat. Removing the primary tumour at this stage has the advantage that it saves the patient from a further major operation at a later date; leaving it alone may, however, be necessary if the patient is very ill due to the effects of the emergency, making it necessary to keep the length and gravity of the operation to the minimum required to save the patient's life.

Tackling the tumour

For many years the standard way of dealing with these emergencies was to embark on a series of three operations. The emergency was dealt with simply by making a temporary colostomy upstream from the site of obstruction or perforation, thus resolving the immediate crisis (by releasing the pent up bowel content or preventing further leakage into the abdomen, respectively). When the patient had recovered sufficiently (several weeks later) the second procedure was performed, aimed at removing the primary tumour and anastomosing (i.e. joining the cut ends of) the bowel again. The third procedure followed a couple of months after that to close the initial colostomy. This came to be regarded as an unnecessarily protracted way of dealing with the problem. Surgeons began to combine stages one and two, or two and three. One reason why the exercise needed to be multi-staged was that the bowel could not be washed out prior to the operation, as would occur before an elective procedure, so that an anastomosis would be in danger of leaking soon after the emergency operation. More recently it has become apparent that in the hands of a suitably experienced surgeon the whole matter can sometimes be dealt with in a single operation, i.e. removal of the affected portion of the bowel (the resection) and anastomosis are carried out without the need for a temporary colostomy. In order to do this the colon upstream from the site of resection is either washed out on the operating table or it is totally removed, the anastomosis being made between the small bowel and the empty colon or rectum on the downstream side of the resection. If the surgeon feels that it is safe to remove the tumour but not to make an anastomosis, the upstream cut end of the colon is brought to the surface as a colostomy, while the other end is closed and returned to the abdomen; a later operation might then be performed to join the ends again, once the patient has recovered from the emergency; this approach is known as Hartmann's procedure.

SURGERY IN THE INCURABLE CASE

Sometimes the surgeon finds, either during preoperative investigation or during operation, that the disease is at a stage at which cure is not possible. This may be because the primary tumour has spread locally to the point at which it cannot be separated from other vital structures around it, or that it has spread via the blood stream to produce widespread secondary tumours, most probably in the liver, which are not surgically curable.

Even if the surgeon is unable to cure the patient, it is usual to try to remove the primary tumour. This is likely to make the patient's remaining life, which may be several years, more comfortable. The surgeon may opt for any of the procedures discussed as curative operations; thus, if the reason for incurability is liver involvement, a standard bowel resection is performed. If the main problem is local advancement, the surgeon is likely to remove the bulk of the primary tumour if this can be achieved safely. Sometimes this is not possible, in which case a colostomy may be required upstream from the tumour to prevent obstruction to the faecal flow.

SURGERY IN THOSE WITH AN HEREDITARY PREDISPOSITION TO BOWEL CANCER

The surgery required in this group of patients has a different set of aims, and hence a rather different technical approach. The details vary with the inherited abnormality and the individual situation. Surgery in these people has two aims—first, to treat a cancer effectively if it has already developed, and secondly, (and more commonly) to try to *prevent* cancer.

Familial adenomatous polyposis (FAP)

As explained earlier (Chapter 6, p. 84), this is a condition in which countless adenomas develop on the lining of the large bowel, usually during the teenage years. When a person is identified as having this condition, so long as cancer has not already occurred, the aims in treatment are as follows:

● to remove the part of the bowel at risk of developing cancer, but at the same time,
● to preserve normal bowel function as far as possible.

Theoretically, the best way to prevent cancer in the colon and rectum affected by FAP is to remove the whole of the large bowel ('total proctocolectomy'). Today, however, this is not regarded by most surgeons as a generally acceptable procedure, as it entails a permanent stoma. Today

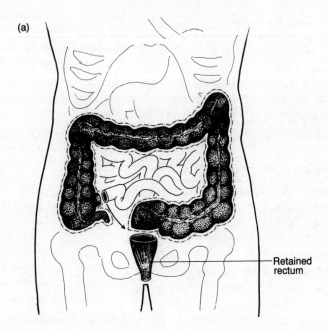

Retained
rectum

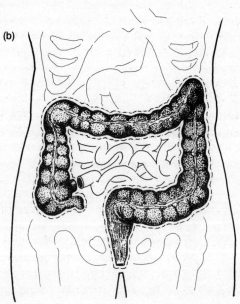

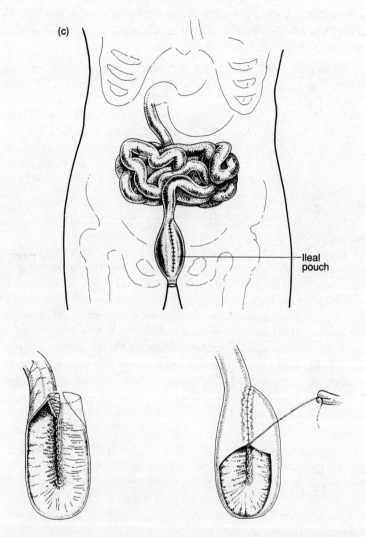

(c)

Ileal pouch

Fig. 14. Alternative operations for FAP. (a) Colectomy and ileorectal ana-stomosis. The colon is removed completely, and the cut end of the small bowel (ileum) is joined to the upper end of the rectum. (b) Restorative proctocolectomy —extent of resection. The whole colon and rectum are removed, leaving the anal canal in place. (c) Restorative proctocolectomy—final result. A 'pouch' of small bowel has been made (inset) and joined to the anal canal to act as a reservoir, which can function much like the removed rectum.

most surgeons would advise one of two alternative operations, both of which have the advantage over total proctocolectomy that the patient continues to pass bowel motions normally:

1. **Colectomy and ileorectal anastomosis.** This operation involves removal of the colon, followed by anastomosis of the ileum (i.e. the small bowel) to the rectum (Fig. 14a). This removes most of the cancer risk but the rectum remains and could go on to develop cancer in the future. The patient therefore requires careful surveillance to try to prevent this (see Chapter 8, p. 145). The operation is usually straightforward, requiring admission to hospital for a period of about two weeks. Preparation, operative technique and aftercare are very much like those applying to anterior resection of the rectum.

2. **Restorative proctocolectomy.** This is a relatively new operation, first used in the late 1970s. It involves complete removal of the colon and rectum (hence removing all cancer risk in the large bowel), but preservation of the anal sphincter mechanism and the fashioning of a new rectum from the lower 30 cm of the ileum (Figs 14b and c). Briefly, the lower ileum is doubled back on itself, in a J configuration, opened up and stitched in a way which produces a 'pouch', or reservoir, which is then sutured to the anus. The pouch is able to store bowel motion prior to its convenient passage. The main problem with this operation is that it can be technically quite demanding, and is more likely to be followed by postoperative complications than colectomy and ileorectal anastomosis. Moreover, although the patient has a lesser cancer risk, careful follow up is nevertheless required to ensure that optimum function of the 'pouch' is maintained.

Occasionally a patient with FAP will have developed cancer already by the time they seek treatment. In this situation, treatment will depend on the site and state of the cancer. If the cancer is in the colon, and at operation it looks as though there is a good chance of cure, the surgeon is likely to perform a colectomy and ileorectal anastomosis, making sure that the cancer is removed radically (see p. 100). If, however, the cancer is in the rectum, the surgeon may opt for a total proctocolectomy, though restorative proctocolectomy is an alternative under suitable circumstances.

Cancer families (see p. 88)

The usual way of dealing with the adenomas in affected family members is to remove them as they are seen at colonoscopy (see p. 80). Sometimes, however, the adenomas are too numerous or too large to be dealt with in this way. Under these circumstances the surgeon may well suggest treatment as in FAP, i.e. colectomy and ileorectal anastomosis with careful postoperative surveillance. Any lumps detected in the ovaries, uterus or breasts will need to be biopsied, and treated as appropriate.

STOMAS—COLOSTOMY AND ILEOSTOMY

A stoma (a Greek word meaning 'mouth') is an artifical opening of the bowel. These days it is brought to the front of the abdomen, though when surgeons first tried to make them around 200 years ago, they were placed at the side or back to avoid the then dangerous step of having to operate directly into the abdominal cavity. Depending on which part of the bowel is brought out to make the stoma, it may be called a 'colostomy' (i.e. a 'colon-stoma') or an 'ileostomy' (i.e. an 'ileum-stoma'). Many people today are under the false impression that 'the treatment of bowel cancer means a bag'. This was never true of all bowel cancers, and today it really is inaccurate. For a start, no one undergoing an attempted curative operation for *colon* cancer needs a permanent stoma, while 50 per cent or less of rectal cancer patients need one.

Types of stoma

There are various types of stoma—a few words of explanation of some of the terms used to describe them are needed first.

Temporary or permanent?
Stomas are made for two main reasons:

1. As a stop-gap, while the bowel starts to recover from a difficult operation or dangerous disease process (e.g. peritonitis or bowel obstruction). In these situations a temporary stoma is made.
2. As a permanent measure, to replace the function of the rectum and anus.

Colostomy or ileostomy?
While most patients who need a stoma as part of the treatment of bowel cancer will have a colostomy, there are some circumstances in which an ileostomy is made instead. For instance, a temporary ileostomy is sometimes made in a patient who has an anastomosis in the transverse or left colon that needs protecting for a while. In rare instances the whole colon

and rectum must be removed, in which case the ileum is the only part of the bowel available to make a permanent stoma.

Loop or terminal stoma?

By and large a temporary stoma is most easily made by bringing the bowel to the abdominal surface through a small opening, holding it there with a plastic or glass rod, rather like a stirrup, and simply opening the bowel. This is known as a 'loop' colostomy or ileostomy, as a loop (a rather misleading word, meaning here simply an undivided length) of bowel has been used. If the stoma is to be permanent after bowel cancer surgery, the cut end, or termination, of the bowel is brought out to the skin surface, hence the name, 'terminal' colostomy.

Conventional or continent?

Usually a stoma is an essentially simple arrangement, with the bowel opening straight onto the skin surface, the owner having no direct control over when the bowel will empty itself. Thus it could be said that the patient is incontinent, though of course the use of a stoma appliance, or bag, keeps everything under satisfactory control. These days, under very limited circumstances, it is possible to make a continent stoma. This may be used in the patient who would otherwise have a conventional *ileostomy* but for whom continence would be a particular desire. This complicated procedure requires the making of a 'pouch' from the lower small bowel to act as a reservoir, with a valve, made from the very end of the small bowel, which prevents the pouch from emptying spontaneously via the ileostomy. The patient is able to empty the pouch by inserting a small plastic tube which passes through the valve, allowing the bowel contents to empty into a plastic jug or into the lavatory. This arrangement, the 'Kock continent ileostomy', is named after the Swedish surgeon who developed it.

Where are stomas sited?

Theoretically a stoma can be sited anywhere on the abdomen, but there are certain general sites which are favoured and a few rules which help to place the stoma optimally within those areas.

Terminal colostomy (see Plate 6)

This type is usually made using the sigmoid colon, so is best placed below the umbilicus, left of the midline (the 'left iliac fossa').

Terminal and loop ileostomies

As the lower end of the ileum, the part used for these stomas, lies in the right iliac fossa, the abdominal wall at this site is favoured.

Loop colostomy

When the transverse colon is used, this type is placed below the ribs on the right side (the right subcostal area); if the sigmoid colon is used, the left iliac fossa is the chosen site.

Choosing the site

It is important that the stoma is located on flat skin, away from bony prominences, scars, and the umbilicus. It needs to pass through a muscle called the rectus abdominis, which runs as a strip down each side of the midline of the abdomen. Moreover, it must be placed where the patient can *see* it, sometimes very difficult in a fat person, in whom the tummy below the umbilicus may be 'over the horizon'. It is almost impossible to gauge accurately where the stoma should be sited when the patient is asleep on the operating table, so it is a very important task *before* an operation in which a stoma is a possibility, to choose very precisely the spot within the area where the stoma is best sited; it is extraordinary how the shape and size of the tummy varies between individuals. Having chosen a likely spot, the stoma care nurse or the doctor will ensure that the site is as satisfactory when the patient stands or sits as it is when lying down. When they are happy that the best spot has been located, they mark it with an indelible pen to guide the surgeon at the operation.

How is a stoma made?

Terminal stoma

The surgeon usually knows at the outset of an operation that a stoma is necessary, though sometimes, perhaps because of unexpected findings, a stoma becomes necessary as the operation progresses. If a stoma is definitely required, the 2–3 cm circular opening in the abdominal wall, sited as outlined above, can be made as the first step in the operation, before the main incision is made. This allows the stomal opening to be made very precisely through the skin, fat, and muscle layers of the abdominal wall, before they are disturbed by the operation proper. This channel is then left alone while the operation proceeds. Towards the end of the operation the cut end of the bowel, with a small clamp applied to it to stop any bowel content contaminating the wound, is delivered through the channel prepared for it in the abdominal wall, and the main abdominal incision is closed. At this point the clamp is removed from the bowel end and a series of fine sutures is inserted to attach the cut end of the bowel to the edges of the circular skin wound. With a colostomy the result is a very simple opening of the bowel end, almost flush with the skin; an ileostomy is constructed slightly differently, in that a small spout, 2–3 cm long, is made by drawing out twice that length of bowel and doubling it back on itself before suturing it to the skin. This ensures that the bowel content is delivered well down into the bag rather than coming out at skin level. This is very important, as the effluent from the ileum is much more irritating to skin than that produced from a colostomy. Having finished making the stoma, a plastic bag appliance is attached to the abdominal wall to enclose the stoma, protecting the skin immediately around the stoma and ready to collect the effluent when it starts to be passed a few days after the operation. Although the plastic bags will be opaque when the stoma has 'settled in', to start with a transparent bag is used to allow the staff to check easily that the stoma remains healthy, with a good blood supply, and so on.

Loop stoma

The decision to make a temporary loop stoma is usually made *during* an operation, so the opening for it has to be made at the end rather than the beginning of the procedure. Whether it is to be placed in the left or right iliac fossa or the right subcostal area (see definitions above) a straight incision is made, about 5–6 cm long, through all layers of the abdominal wall. The chosen loop of bowel is brought through the opening, and supported at skin level by a plastic or glass rod. The bowel is then opened and the cut edges stitched to the skin. A bag appliance is attached as for a terminal stoma.

POSTOPERATIVE RECOVERY

Introduction

These days elective surgery for bowel cancer is much safer than it used to be. Nevertheless around 2–5 per cent of patients may die in the first month after the operation and rather more will suffer complications of varying seriousness. To keep things as safe as possible, the nursing and medical staff have a routine set of procedures which unsuspecting patients and their visitors may find baffling.

Tubes, drains, and bags

On return to the ward there will be several tubes or other appliances attached to the patient for various reasons. There will be an intravenous drip running via a tube attached to the arm or the side of the neck. Through this the patient will receive around three litres of fluid per 24 hours in place of the normal intake by mouth (eating will not resume until the bowel begins to work, usually a few days after the operation). The fluid volume and composition is reviewed each day by the doctors; it must compensate for the fluid lost as urine (1.5 litres), in the breath (500 ml), perspiration (500 ml) and any abnormal losses, such as via drainage tubes. If the patient needs blood this will be given via the drip, and it is also a convenient route for the administration of certain drugs, such as antibiotics. Another tube, and one which is very obvious to the patient if it is present, is the nasogastric tube, passing through the nose and down into the stomach. This is used to drain away the digestive juices which are not required and which may cause nausea and even vomiting if they build up excessively. However, many surgeons have found that this tube, which can be rather uncomfortable and intrusive, is not routinely necessary and have dispensed with it. In addition, the bladder will be emptying via a catheter which drains into a bag. This makes it possible to keep an eye on the volume of urine being produced, hence helping with fluid prescription; it also relieves the patient of the need to get out of bed to pass urine in the first few postoperative days. There may be drainage tubes running from the abdomen to remove any fluid or blood which may collect around the site of the operation; draining them away helps to prevent infections and leakage from the anastomosis. These drains may be in the form of tubes, in which case they will empty into a bag or a suction pump at the side of the bed, or they may be strips of soft plastic or rubber, the end of which will be surrounded by a dressing or a bag on the tummy wall to collect the fluid. Drains usually remain in place for around 2–4 days, though in some circumstances they will be required for a longer period. The final encumbrance, if present, will be a stoma appliance, a plastic bag to collect bowel contents if the formation of a stoma has been necessary. To start with this will produce no discharge, but within a few days the bowel should start to act; the nurses will look after it completely to start with,

but as the patient recovers he or she will be trained in its care. This will
be dealt with in more detail in Chapter 9 (see p. 145)

Medication

Infections, in particular in the wound, are kept to a minimum these days
by the use of antibiotics given for a short period around the time of the
operation. The first dose is usually given via the intravenous drip at the
beginning of the operation; two more doses are given by the same route
in the first 24 hours after operation.

Pain relieving drugs (analgesics) will be required during recovery.
Their obvious aim is to diminish discomfort, but in addition they make
breathing and movement easier, thereby decreasing the risk of chest and
other complications. Initially they may be given as an injection into a
muscle—the buttock or thigh (i.e. an intramuscular injection)—which
allows rapid absorption into the bloodstream. Sometimes they are
administered as a continuous injection via a small needle placed under
the skin of the arm, held in place with sticking plaster; a small pump
attached to the needle via a thin tube injects a graduated amount of the
analgesic continuously, offering more satisfactory pain relief than intermittent intramuscular injections. When the patient begins to take fluids
by mouth a few days after the operation, analgesia is usually taken by
mouth instead.

Diet

Food intake stops for a few days after this type of surgery as the gastrointestinal tract cannot transmit or digest it. Lack of food does not matter
for a short period, but as soon as the bowel shows signs of working, the
patient will be offered small amounts of water and other drinks to start
with, soon followed by progression to a light diet and then on to normal
food intake within 5–6 days after the operation. There are no particular
dietary needs or restrictions after bowel cancer surgery, except for a few
minor rules for some patients with a stoma; more of this later.

Discussion of outcome

When the patient has recovered sufficiently, the surgeon will discuss
what has been done and what the future is likely to hold. If all has gone
well the patient and relatives will be reassured at an early stage, usually

within 24 hours or so of the operation. The surgeon will not be in a position to give a full account of the outlook until the pathologist has been able to complete the examination of the operation specimen; this takes several days, perhaps up to a week sometimes. Patients and their families differ in the amount of information that they wish to receive from the surgeon. They will need to know about how long recovery from the operation is likely to take and will want to know about the functional outcome—the effects on bowel activity, stomas, etc. But most important is the chance of cure. The surgeon, armed with the pathologist's report, should be able to tell the patient the Dukes' stage of the tumour (see p. 35), i.e. the pathological stage of advancement, and this will give a good idea of the percentage chance that the patient is cured. In addition, the surgeon may have evidence from the operation indicating that the patient is not curable; this information must be imparted with great care, usually after careful explanation and consultation with the relatives, who play a central role in helping the patient to understand and deal with the information. They may feel that the patient should not be told the full story in these circumstances; the surgeon will certainly take these feelings fully into account though the patient's right to know must also always be in the surgeon's mind. The whole problem of imparting information and discussing its implications with patients and their families is one of great complexity sometimes. Despite the best intentions and efforts of the staff, however, patients and relatives may be confused by the barrage of technicalities directed at them; if this is the case, they should always feel free to ask to see the doctors again, including the consultant, to discuss things further.

Getting up and about

Lying inert in bed after major surgery predisposes the patient to various complications, including chest infection, blood clots, and bed sores. An important part of postoperative care, therefore, is early encouragement to move. Initially this will entail breathing exercises and active leg movements, but within a day or two the patient will be encouraged to get out of bed to take short walks, aided by the nurses; sitting crumpled and inert in a bedside chair is *not* a good alternative.

Care of the operation wound

Unless there is a stoma, the only part of the surgeon's handiwork visible to the patient is the skin wound, closed either with conventional stitches or small metal clips. If all goes well, the skin is sufficiently well healed for the stitches or clips to be removed about ten days after the operation. This is a simple and, surprisingly for most, a pain-free procedure, carried out by a nurse either in a side ward reserved for such activities or on the patient's bed in the main ward.

General state

The experience of having gone through a major operation is an enormous and hopefully unusual event in one's life. Most people find the train of events very tiring and often depressing. What seemed like parts of life which could be taken for granted become mountainously difficult for a while—breathing, coughing, and laughing may hurt, a drink of water becomes a longed for luxury, standing straight and walking may seem impossible. Privacy is lost and dignity diminished. Hopefully the doctors, nurses, and others around in the postoperative period will understand and help to deal with these aspects of the road to recovery. Meanwhile, it is important for the patient and their family to know that this period of frustration and struggle is common to all following major surgery, whatever the reason for the operation, and that with sympathetic support, what seems like interminable discomfort and strife is usually rewarded by complete return to effortless coping with the routines of life.

GOING HOME AFTER SURGERY

Following any major surgery it is usual for the patient to stay in hospital until after removal of skin stitches on about the tenth postoperative day. By then they are taking a normal diet, the bowel is functioning fairly normally and they are able to get about. If there is a stoma, the patient will be in the process of learning how to look after it by the tenth day, but will usually need to stay in for a few more days while they consolidate their skills. The nurses will have checked on the home situation prior to discharge to make sure that the family are able to cope with someone still unable to fend for themselves. If the patient lives alone, especially if elderly, or has a stoma, special arrangements will be made, perhaps including calls by the district nurse or the stoma care nurse, or an initial period of convalescence.

8
Other treatments: radiotherapy, chemotherapy, immunotherapy, and lasers

Unlike some other types of malignant disease, bowel cancer is a condition in which surgery is still by far the most important form of treatment. However, surgery is an anatomically circumscribed treatment, so that its use in a disease in which microscopic spread may be present around the primary tumour, as well as in other parts of the body, is frequently followed by recurrence. It is for this reason that doctors and scientists have searched for other treatments, either to supplant surgery completely or, in the shorter term, to be added to surgery to enhance its results.

Radiotherapy (the delivering of X-ray and other types of energy beam), chemotherapy (the use of cancer-killing drugs), and immunotherapy (the enhancement of the body's natural anti-cancer defences) all offer some hope of improving the outcome in bowel cancer. Much research effort has gone into defining the effects on the disease, and to making the treatments safer and more comfortable for the patient. So far, we have quite good evidence that some forms of treatment decrease the risk of recurrence of cancer around the site of removal of a rectal cancer. As far as improvement in survival is concerned (i.e. curing patients who might otherwise have succumbed to the disease), this has been more difficult to prove. But there are good reasons for optimism today, as new techniques and methods of treatment give hope for demonstrable survival improvement.

RADIOTHERAPY

Radiotherapy involves the delivery of high energy rays or other forms of radioactivity which seriously damage the cancer cells, leading to their destruction over the ensuing weeks. Radiotherapy may be delivered by:

- 'external beam', from a large machine under which the patient lies to receive treatment;

- 'intraluminal beam', using a machine passed into the rectum to press against the tumour, or;
- 'wire implant', in which radioactive wires are inserted temporarily into the tumour.

Basically, radiotherapy may be used in any of three roles in bowel cancer, as:

- *adjuvant therapy*—additional treatment to radical surgery;
- *primary treatment*, i.e., as a curative treatment, instead of surgery, or;
- *palliative treatment* to relieve the symptoms of incurable disease.

Adjuvant therapy

The aim of adjuvant radiotherapy is to kill cancer cells not dealt with by the surgeon. As radiotherapy aimed at the colon is more likely to damage surrounding organs, especially the small bowel, adjuvant radiotherapy is used mainly in the management of rectal tumours, where such damage is easier to avoid.

Much research has gone into evaluating adjuvant radiotherapy over the past two decades. It may be given before or after the operation; there are even some doctors looking at its use before *and* after surgery (the so-called 'sandwich' technique). In a few centres, especially in the US, radiotherapy is given *during* surgery, allowing a large dose to be directed very precisely at the area from which the tumour has just been removed. This may have the advantage of high dose treatment with minimum risk of damage to other organs.

The usefulness of adjuvant radiotherapy remains controversial amongst cancer specialists. At present few would dispute its role in the patient with a large rectal cancer in whom it is likely that surgery may leave some of the tumour behind. It is with the average-sized tumour that radiotherapy remains debatable. Preoperative radiotherapy has been shown to decrease the size of the primary tumour which may make subsequent surgery more effective; it probably also has the effect of destroying tumour tissue which is growing in the lymph nodes. It seems that radiotherapy, especially when given *after* surgery, probably decreases the risk of recurrence in the pelvis, but the improvement in chance of cure appears to be small using the presently available technology. Nevertheless, research continues to try to improve this form of treatment and to define its exact role.

Primary treatment

The bowel cancers most amenable to treatment using radiotherapy alone are small, superficial tumours in the lower part of the rectum — a few per cent of all cases. Broadly these are the same tumours which can be dealt with by the local excision operation (see p. 111), i.e. they are sufficiently small and apparently sufficiently localized that a major operation to remove a large volume of tissue is not required.

One possible disadvantage of radical radiotherapy rather than local excision for these small tumours is that the pathologist is not able to receive and examine the whole tumour; thus a full appraisal of the chances of recurrence is not possible. However, in some cases, particularly if the patient's general health is poor, the main priority may be to avoid an operation altogether; it is in these circumstances that this approach may be most appropriate.

Sometimes radiotherapy is used in an attempt to cure a patient with a larger tumour, who is unfit (perhaps because of heart or lung disease) for the appropriate major surgery. Under these circumstances the radiotherapist will be consulted in the hope that radical radiotherapy will destroy the primary tumour and its lymphatic drainage—a surgical operation without the knife! In such a case it is likely that the tumour will be greatly diminished in volume rather than cured, but sometimes the tumour does disappear, with a long-term prospect of cure.

Palliative treatment

For the patient with an incurable rectal tumour, either as an initially inoperable cancer, or as one that has recurred after the primary operation, radiotherapy may be used to alleviate symptoms. Pain due to spread of the tumour to the muscles, nerves, and bones of the pelvis can be severe. Patients may suffer unbearable feelings of 'fullness' or other odd sensations in the pelvic region, possibly due to involvement of the pelvic nerves. Radiotherapy is particularly useful in helping to control these symptoms.

Planning treatment

Under any of the circumstances described above the patient will first visit the consultant radiotherapist for an initial examination to assess the suitability for radiotherapy, and to choose which form of therapy is most appropriate. If the radiotherapist agrees that treatment is worthwhile, a planning session will be arranged at which X-ray examination, perhaps including a body scan, will be performed. This produces a simulation of active radiotherapy treatment; it gives a detailed picture of the anatomy of the area to be treated (this differs between patients), helping the radiotherapist to calculate the exact dose to be delivered, and if beam therapy is to be applied, the direction and size of the beams to be used and the 'fractionation', i.e. the division of the treatment into daily doses. This process will ensure that the maximum possible benefit is achieved from treatment.

Receiving radiotherapy

The procedure differs depending on the form of therapy chosen.

External beam therapy

Radiotherapy is usually given on weekdays only, allowing both patients and staff a rest at weekends. The treatment is given by radiographers (i.e. the people directly controlling the X-ray machines) under the direction of the radiotherapist (the doctor who plans the therapy). External beam therapy is applied in special rooms, shielded to prevent passage of the treatment beams beyond their walls. The patient lies on a table for treatment, and once made comfortable, will be left alone in the room, so that the radiographers do not receive the treatment as well. However, they are just outside, watching the patient by closed-circuit television and in constant two-way voice contact by intercom. Each treatment lasts no more than a few minutes.

   Depending on the size of dose to be applied, the patient may need to attend just once or up to 25–30 times, spread over 4–6 weeks. This may be done as an out-patient though in some cases, for medical or social reasons, the patient may be admitted to hospital for the duration of the treatment.

Intraluminal therapy

This is an unusual form of treatment in the UK, though it is more widely used in the US and in continental Europe. As with external beam therapy, treatment may be spread over several visits, though not for so long a period. Instead of the patient lying on a table, they are placed in the 'knee/elbow' position, in which they crouch, face downwards, with the bottom upwards, their weight taken on the knees and lower legs, and elbows and forearms. The instrument which delivers the beam is inserted, like a sigmoidoscope, through the anus so that the end comes to lie against the tumour.

Wire implant therapy

Particularly careful planning is required for this form of treatment, which is sometimes known as 'brachytherapy'. The aim is to place a series of radioactive wires, usually made of iridium, into the tumour, where they release radioactivity very precisely, with a lesser risk of surrounding damage. In order that the wires are placed exactly, and to prevent their movement during irradiation, they may be inserted using a special frame, or template, attached to the perineum (the skin area around the anus), with the patient under general anaesthesia during insertion. The patient has to remain in hospital during the 2–8 days that the wires remain in place; if a template is used they must remain in bed, so that the wires are not displaced. During the period of treatment, the patient effectively becomes mildly radioactive, so they must remain in a single occupancy room with restriction on visiting—children and pregnant women will not be allowed to come into close proximity as they are at a greater risk from the effects of radiation. As soon as the implant is removed, these risks disappear completely: the patient does not remain radioactive!

Side-effects

As with any form of treatment, radiotherapy can have side-effects. These may occur during or immediately after treatment, or may not develop for months or even years. They range from the merely uncomfortable or inconvenient to the far less frequent severely incapacitating. It may seem as you read this section that it all seems too much. But remember that these side-effects are being listed to provide some insight should they occur, and that merely listing them makes it appear that everyone experiences them. This is, of course, not the case, and it is difficult to write at length about the experience of *not* getting side-effects!

Early side-effects

Skin reactions The commonest problems are soreness of the skin caused by the beam as it passes through to reach the target. Usually these reactions are no worse than something akin to mild sunburn, but they can be more severe, in rare cases leading to destruction ('necrosis')

of the skin. Mild reactions may need no treatment, or a soothing oint-
ment may be applied. More severe reactions may require a rest from
radiotherapy.

Bowel upsets   Radiation has its main effect on rapidly reproducing cells
(tumour cells have this characteristic, hence their sensitivity to this form
of treatment). The mucosal lining of the intestine is also composed of
rapidly dividing cells, so it, too, is rather sensitive to irradiation. The
rectum itself or any segments of small bowel 'in the line of fire' may
become inflamed during therapy, leading to symptoms mimicking gastroenteritis, or a 'tummy upset'. This usually responds to antidiarrhoeal
medication; sometimes treatment may have to be modified to deal with
this problem.

Later reactions

First of all it should be said that late effects of radiation for rectal cancer
are uncommon and usually not severe; sometimes, however, they are
incapacitating, or even life-threatening. It may seem odd that reactions
can occur long after treatment has finished. Probably what happens is
that the radiation has an effect on the minute blood vessels in the organ
affected, leading to a gradual deterioration in its blood supply. This has a
different effect depending on the organ involved.

Rectum   Radiation damage may produce transient symptoms, though
often they are longer lasting and low grade. It causes diarrhoea, mucous
discharge and the passage of blood. Treatment is relatively difficult,
mainly involving supportive treatment with antidiarrhoeal drugs, blood
transfusion, etc., while waiting for the symptoms to remit. Treatment
with steroid enemas may be given, though the usefulness of this treatment is debatable.

   More seriously, the rectal wall may be sufficiently weakened that it
gives way, causing faeces to leak into the vagina in women, or the
bladder in men (in each case the organ directly in front of the rectum is
affected, see Fig. 6, p. 14). This complication is uncommon, requiring
major surgery to deal with it.

Bladder   Bladder injury is characterized by a frequent desire to pass
urine, including at night, and the passage of blood. In the same way that
the rectum can leak, so too can the bladder; in women this leads to the
passage of urine from the vagina. As with rectal fistula, this calls for
major surgery.

Small intestine   This is potentially the most serious radiation-induced injury. The small bowel is most likely to be damaged if *postoperative* radiotherapy is given: the small intestine sometimes adheres to the front of the rectum after surgery, thus holding it directly in the path of the beam. The intestine may become narrowed ('stenotic'), causing severe cramping pains due to partial obstruction or, if severe enough, complete obstruction of the bowel. Alternatively the damaged bowel can perforate causing peritonitis. The bowel may perforate into another organ, such as the bladder or the rectum, producing a fistula, and leakage of small intestinal content into the involved organ.

CHEMOTHERAPY

Chemotherapy is treatment using drugs which attack cancer cells; there are many types of drug available, but they all act either by killing the cancer cells outright or by disabling them so that they cannot reproduce themselves; therefore, as they age and die, they have not produced fresh cancer cells to replace them. Chemotherapy may be given in bowel cancer either as adjuvant therapy to try to increase the chances that surgery will be curative, or as palliative treatment, to try to minimize the symptoms due to incurable cancer. At the moment it is not possible to use chemotherapy alone to try to achieve a cure for bowel cancer, though this is possible in some other sorts of tumour, such as some in childhood, some testicular tumours, and lymphomas.

Adjuvant therapy

As with radiotherapy, drugs can be given around the time of radical surgery in the hope that this will improve the chance of cure (adjuvant therapy). Until quite recently there has been little evidence that chemo-therapy given in this way had much effect on the outcome in bowel cancer; in the last few years, however, there has been emerging evidence that certain combinations of chemotherapy drugs may have a more useful effect than was seen previously using single drugs. Adjuvant chemotherapy has been looked at using two main methods of adminis-tration: systemic therapy, i.e. giving the drug into the general blood circulation, and local therapy, i.e. directed very specifically at the site expected to benefit from the drug.

Systemic therapy

Drugs may be given either into the bloodstream or by mouth, to be absorbed into the bloodstream from the intestine. Either way the drug is then carried to all parts of the body. Most chemotherapy drugs 'attack' any very actively replicating cells; as cancer cells are particularly active in this regard, they are most vigorously attacked. The problem with this form of therapy is that other rapidly dividing cells, such as normal blood-making cells and those cells lining the normal intestine, are also affected by chemotherapy, causing anaemia, decreased defence against infection, nausea, vomiting and diarrhoea. Temporary hair loss is sometimes a side-effect of chemotherapy, but not very frequently with the drugs used in bowel cancer. Side-effects can usually be minimized, but if the treat-ment is to have its full effect some unwanted effects are fairly likely.

The drug used most frequently in bowel cancer patients is called 5-fluorouracil (or 5-FU). Although more active in bowel cancer than any other chemotherapy agents, even this one has not been found to show any major effect until quite recently. A review of the overall effect on survival suggested that it might improve the proportion of patients surviving for five years by up to 4 per cent. Results from trials carried out in the US have been published in the past year which suggest that in some colon cancer patients at least, it may have an important role as an adjuvant agent when used in combination with a drug called Levamisole. This drug has been available for many years for the treatment of worm infestations, and was known to have a mildly stimulating effect on the body's defence system, i.e. it is an 'immuno-stimulant'. American doctors and scientists have produced evidence that suggests that some patients with Dukes' stage C colon cancer may be prevented from devel-oping recurrent disease by undergoing one year of intermittent 5-FU and Levamisole therapy. It is too early to be sure of this effect or to know whether the effect, if it truly exists, will benefit other patient groups.

If 5-FU is given intravenously the patient must be admitted to hospital; the drug is then given either as a continuous infusion via a drip in the arm or as a series of 'bolus' injections (i.e. doses given by syringe injection). Usually treatment is given as a series of 'courses', with rest periods between. The blood is regularly checked to monitor the effect on blood cells; anaemia may require blood transfusion, while a marked decrease in the white cells, which protect against infection, may require treatment with antibiotics.

Local therapy

Because of the unwanted side-effects of systemic therapy, and in order to allow higher concentrations of the drug to be directed at the diseased area, local therapy has been developed which aims to confine the drug mainly to the area containing the cancer tissue. The liver is the organ in which local therapy has been tried in cases of bowel cancer, in order to treat or try to prevent secondary tumours.

Intra-arterial therapy   Although it requires an operation, it is possible to place a small tube in the main artery to the liver, and to inject the drug at a constant rate, either using a pump outside or inside the body. The 'inside pump' has the major advantage that the patient is not attached to any equipment, and is free to leave hospital once the pump has been inserted and set running, and they have recovered from the operation. The patient visits the hospital to check the action of the pump and to have it topped up with the drug, via a needle passed through the skin into the pump.

As yet the evidence that this expensive form of therapy has any very useful effect on the disease is rather weak. Studies in the US suggest that it can cause the tumour in the liver to shrink, but the improvement in well-being of the patient and the degree of prolongation of life have not been measured adequately. A well-designed trial in which some patients, randomly chosen, receive this treatment while others do not, is in progress in the UK.

Portal perfusion   Another approach to local therapy is its use in the adjuvant setting. As the liver is the commonest site of further disease after surgery for bowel cancer, researchers tried giving chemotherapy via the vein that takes blood (and cancer cells) from the bowel to the liver— the portal vein (see Fig. 4, p. 10). The technique requires the insertion of a tube into the portal vein during the operation to remove the primary bowel tumour, *in patients in whom the liver appears to be free of cancer*. 5-FU is then given by slow infusion over the ensuing week in the hope that any cells which might have spread to the liver, and which might later grow into detectable secondary cancers, are killed before they can do any harm. Results from several trials in which the outcome in patients receiving or not receiving this treatment were compared, have given preliminary evidence that this approach may have the effect hoped for, at

least in certain subgroups of patients. Further trials are in progress to try
to confirm these early pointers.

Palliative therapy

Patients with advanced disease, especially if the liver is involved and the
patient is suffering severe symptoms, are sometimes given 5-FU in the
hope that it will shrink the tumour sufficiently to diminish symptoms.
Again there is recent information to suggest that 5-FU in combination
with another drug—this time folinic acid—may work to greater effect.

COMBINED RADIOTHERAPY AND CHEMOTHERAPY

Although the results of adjuvant radiotherapy and chemotherapy have
been relatively disappointing in terms of survival improvement following
surgery for bowel cancer, there is the theoretical possibility that, given
together, they might have a more promising effect, especially in rectal
cancer. It might be that radiotherapy would decrease the risk of local
recurrence in the pelvis, while chemotherapy might help to prevent
distant metastasis, the overall additive effect being lives saved. There are
some promising results from small treatment trials in the US to suggest
that this may be so, and a large-scale trial in the UK is looking at radiotherapy and portal perfusion of 5-FU given separately or together. It will
be some time before we see the results of this experimental approach.

IMMUNOTHERAPY

The human body, like all living things, is able to recognize 'foreign'
invaders and make some attempt to kill or remove them. Thus the body
mounts an attack on germs, transplanted tissues (including transfused
blood), splinters or thorns in the skin, and cancers. Unfortunately the
response to some invaders, such as certain germs and many cancers, is
inadequate, so that the body is overwhelmed. It is quite possible, even
likely, that the body frequently manages to kill very small cancers
without us even knowing that anything has happened. But with cancers
large enough to be detectable the response has already failed, thus
allowing the cancer to grow to the detectable size.

Immunotherapy aims to strengthen or reinforce the body's own defences against cancer. Various agents, such as BCG, a very mild form of tuberculosis germ, either alone or with chemotherapy agents, have been tried in advanced bowel cancer, but so far with little obvious success. As mentioned above, the results of the studies using Levamisole have been published in preliminary form, suggesting that this immuno-stimulant may have a useful adjuvant effect when used with 5-FU; used by itself, however, it has not been shown to be useful in bowel cancer patients.

Another approach which comes under the banner of immunotherapy is the application of drugs known as 'biological response modifiers'. These very expensive drugs very specifically enhance the effectiveness of the body's natural cellular defences against cancer. This approach is at a very experimental phase at present, but is an area which may hold promise for the future in bowel cancer.

Yet another promising variation on the immunotherapy theme is the application of monoclonal antibodies, allowing so-called 'targeted therapy'.

Targeted therapy

Using monoclonal antibodies, attempts are being made to use immune recognition to 'target' tumours. The body naturally produces proteins called antibodies which recognize and attach themselves to foreign proteins, known as antigens, in germs, cancers, etc. Each antigen stimulates the production of its corresponding antibody.

In the past few years, scientists have developed a way of producing very pure forms of antibody, the so-called monoclonal antibodies (MAbs). When certain MAbs are injected into the bloodstream they attach themselves to an antigen within a cancer which they recognize as 'their' antigen. By chemically attaching a radioisotope to the MAb, pictures of the cancer, with the MAb/isotope complex attached to it, can be taken using a gamma camera. If a stronger isotope or a chemotherapy drug is attached to the MAb, these substances can damage the cancer cells once they have arrived at their target.

At present, a major problem with this approach is that the MAbs are not sufficiently specific for the cancer antigens, so they tend to become attached also, though to a much lesser extent, to normal cells. This would mean that targeted therapy would damage normal tissues as well as the cancer cells. So work continues to refine this new tool in the hope that monoclonal antibody targeted therapy will allow more effective attack on metastatic (i.e. distantly spread) cancer, than is possible by any presently available means.

LASERS

Lasers have assumed an almost mythical status amongst many people, who seem to believe that they can cure where more conventional approaches have failed. At present, in bowel cancer at least, reality falls far short of the myth. The laser works by delivering large amounts of energy very precisely in the form of light. When applied to a tumour, or any other tissue, it causes vaporization or simple killing of tumour tissue by high temperature.

This 'high-tech' approach has been used in some cases of advanced rectal cancer to try to relieve obstruction, and in some rectal cancer patients not fit for general anaesthesia and conventional surgery. The laser instrument is passed through the anus and 'fired' directly at the surface of the tumour. It is a purely local therapy, having no role as yet in the management of widespread disease. As with any treatment it has its complications—the risk of perforation of the bowel, bleeding from the tumour, or failure to control the disease, all limit its present usefulness.

9
After-care

When initial treatment has finished, regular checks on progress will be made by the hospital doctors—this is known as 'follow-up'. Some patients will need the continuing support of a stoma care nurse, while others will need the constant availability of those who specialize in helping the terminally ill.

WHAT IS FOLLOW-UP?

In those in whom treatment has been potentially curative, follow-up has several purposes:

- it allows the surgeon to check for the development of recurrent cancer;
- if metachronous tumours (i.e. *new* primary bowel cancers) occur these can be identified and dealt with;
- the patient may feel assured by regular contact with the surgeon, having the opportunity to discuss any worries related to their previous illness;
- the surgeon, by following up all his or her cancer patients, has the opportunity to check that the results obtained are as good as might realistically be expected. This is known as 'surgical audit'.

WHAT ARE THEY LOOKING FOR?

Local recurrence

As discussed earlier, the margin of clearance of a rectal cancer may be less than that achievable in a colon cancer. Correspondingly, rectal cancer patients are at a greater risk of developing tumour recurrence in the pelvis, at the site of the primary tumour—so-called 'local' recurrence.

Distant recurrence

The commonest site of distant recurrence due to spread via the blood-stream is the liver; less commonly the lungs, bones, or other organs may be involved.

New cancers

As mentioned above, about 1 in 20–30 patients will develop a new colorectal cancer at a later date. In many others the benign forerunners of cancers, adenomas, will grow anew. New tumours, benign or malignant, can occur anywhere along the length of the remaining large bowel, though they are more likely to grow in the rectum and sigmoid colon (if still present).

Non-cancer problems

Imperfect healing of the operation scar may manifest itself as small areas of infection around stitches beneath the skin; part or all of the scar may be weak, leading to a hernia, especially if there has been a wound infection in the immediate postoperative period. The patient may have worries about their health, their work, and their family in the aftermath of their cancer. They may want to discuss these problems with the surgeon, who must be on the look out for the worried patient trying to cover it up, or trying 'not to bother the doctor'. Much of the point of follow-up is missed if these aspects of postoperative care are ignored or skimped.

HOW OFTEN SHOULD FOLLOW-UP VISITS OCCUR?

Most surgeons see their follow-up patients 3–6 monthly during the first 2 or 3 years, when the risk of recurrence is at its greatest; around 80 per cent of recurrences will become apparent during this period. Thereafter the visits become less frequent, perhaps 6–12 monthly.

HOW IS IT DONE?

There is enormous variation in the way different surgeons follow-up their patients, depending on the individual surgeon's perception of the usefulness of particular procedures and of follow-up in general.

Clinical examination

The follow-up visit will normally begin with a few questions about general health, together with more specific ones about bowel function, aches and pains, etc. The surgeon will want to carry out a general examination, concentrating on the abdomen, feeling for any lumps, especially in the liver, and checking the healing of the operation scar. In rectal cancer patients in particular, the rectum will be reviewed by examination with the gloved index finger of the surgeon, and by direct inspection with a sigmoidoscope; these steps will allow the surgeon to check for any lumps that may have grown in the pelvis outside or inside the rectum.

Blood tests

In the early period after surgery the surgeon may want to check for anaemia with a simple blood count. They may also check the blood for 'tumour markers'.

Tumour markers

This is a complicated and controversial subject. Tumour markers are substances released into the bloodstream which, if found, suggest that the patient has developed recurrence or a new primary cancer. Theoretically this sounds very useful: in practice it's not so simple.

What are they? These substances are produced by cancer cells; theoretically, the most useful ones would be those which are *only* produced by tumour cells and not by normal cells, so that if *any* of the substance is found in the blood it would be a highly specific indicator of trouble. But in practice there are no 'tumour-specific' markers for bowel cancer; what we have instead are 'tumour associated' markers, produced mainly by bowel cancer cells, but to a lesser extent by other types of cancer, the diseased bowel in other, non-malignant bowel conditions and even, in small amounts, by perfectly normal bowel tissue. The most widely known tumour marker in bowel cancer is carcinoembryonic antigen— CEA for short.

How useful is CEA? The CEA level in the bloodstream rises above the normal low level *before*, or at the same time as, symptoms develop in around 75 per cent of those in which recurrent tumours grow. One of

the problems with tumour markers however, and CEA in particular, is
that the amount found in the blood is related to the volume of tumour
present to release the marker substance. Very frequently the amount of
the marker in the blood will only reach suspicious levels when the
recurrent tumour has reached untreatable proportions, usually within
the liver.

So what use are *tumour markers?*   There has been a lot of research over
the past 15 years on the use of regular blood sampling to check CEA
levels, in order to allow early diagnosis and treatment of recurrence. It
has yet to be proven, however, that this intensive approach, requiring
monthly visits for blood tests, improves the outlook for patients. Does
early treatment improve the outlook for those few in which treatment is
still possible? Or is it true, as one American cancer expert has said, that
'. . . the only product [of regular CEA monitoring] for most patients is
the needless anxiety produced by the premature knowledge of the
presence of a fatal disease'? Research continues to assess the role of
regular blood tests for tumour markers and to develop new ones; meanwhile some surgeons use the test, while most do not.

Endoscopy

The most sensitive way of checking the lining of the bowel for the
growth of new benign or malignant tumours is colonoscopy. This technique also allows the surgeon to check for recurrence in the colon,
beyond the reach of the short out-patient sigmoidoscope. Some surgeons,
therefore, advocate regular (usually 3-yearly) colonoscopy. However,
most recurrent tumours develop *outside* the bowel, and are therefore not
visible by endoscopy.

X-rays and scans

Barium enema is less sensitive than colonoscopy for detecting small
adenomas in the bowel. If the surgeon without easy access to a colonoscope wants to carry out a routine check, barium enema is the preferred
method. The liver, and to a lesser extent, the rest of the abdomen, are
difficult to check for recurrence simply by out-patient examination by
the surgeon. Computerized axial tomography (CAT or CT) scanning
is a sensitive technique for the detection of recurrence in these sites;
ultrasound scanning is an alternative, cheaper, and less sensitive method

in this context. Some surgeons advocate regular scanning as part of follow-up.

WHEN DOES FOLLOW-UP STOP?

Many surgeons feel that the advantages of follow-up after 5 years are very small as the period of greatest risk has passed; at this stage, therefore, patients will often be told that the chances of further problems are minimal and follow-up will be stopped.

WHY BOTHER WITH FOLLOW-UP?

Although the foregoing sounds perfectly sensible and humane, there are some who would argue with the whole basis of follow-up as routinely practised. Let's look at why this might be, by going through the list of reasons why follow-up might seem 'a good thing', as laid out at the beginning of this chapter:

● **Recurrence detection.** The great majority of recurrent tumours produce symptoms *between* follow-up visits, alerting the patient to the need to seek medical advice. So some doctors argue that routine follow-up to detect recurrence could be dispensed with simply by telling the patient to return if they develop certain symptoms, which could be explained to them at the outset.

● **New bowel tumour detection.** There is a 3–5 per cent risk that the average bowel cancer patient will develop a new primary tumour (rather than a recurrence due to the previous primary tumour). In order to detect this small group, vastly greater numbers who will never have this problem have to be put through regular, quite expensive and invasive tests; and this rather intensive method of detection would only be useful if early detection were of real benefit to the individual patient.

● **Patient reassurance.** It could be argued that, rather than reassuring patients by examining them regularly, the surgeon might actually make matters worse by reminding them constantly of the risk of further problems rather than letting them get on with their lives.

● **Surgical audit.** Surgeons always need to review their own performance by keeping in touch with new developments in practice in other institutions, but also by being self-critical and eager to maintain a high standard in the management of every case. This is aided by knowing, for instance, how often their cancer patients develop recurrent tumours, what their expectation of cure is, and the frequency of other postoperative problems. This demands regular follow-up visits with very careful record keeping. In practice most surgeons are rushed off their feet simply keeping up with treating patients; often there just isn't time to use follow-up in this highly desirable way. But without careful audit much of the benefit of follow-up is lost.

These arguments for and against regular follow-up visits are important. Some would say that if surgeons simply shook hands, gave a little advice about returning if symptoms developed and waved goodbye to patients after surgery, the chaos of the average out-patient clinic might be diminished and those patients presenting for the first time with new problems would be seen that much quicker. But most surgeons do, however, feel that follow-up is useful, and see their postoperative patients for a few years at least, until the risk of recurrent disease has greatly diminished.

FOLLOW-UP IN THE HEREDITARY CONDITIONS

Follow-up of individuals and families carrying a genetic prediposition to bowel cancer requires a different approach and organization. Medical attendants have two broad responsibilities in these cases:

(1) to offer continuing care for the individuals, and;
(2) to offer advice and support to the whole family.

In order to fulfil both functions, registries have a major part to play. A registry records details of the known family members, their health and treatment, and helps to ensure that individual family members are kept aware of new information regarding the disease, through the doctor looking after them, and that they are contacted if they miss any follow-up appointments. Without this backup it would be easy for doctors to lose track of family members, perhaps leading to avoidable tragedies.

Familial adenomatous polyposis (FAP)

Follow-up in FAP families includes regular checking of the teenagers to see whether they have developed polyps, and the examination of those who have undergone surgery.

Pre-diagnosis follow-up

If a child has been found to be free of polyps, the usual plan is to see them yearly to examine the rectum using a sigmoidoscope. This simple out-patient procedure is all that is required in these circumstances. This arrangement usually continues until about age 35 unless polyps are seen one day, in which case surgery will be offered (see p. 115).

Postoperative follow-up

The person who has undergone surgery for FAP (see p. 115) is seen 6 monthly if a colectomy and ileorectal anastomosis has been performed. This allows the surgeon to keep a regular eye on the rectal lining, so that if any large polyps appear or if the smaller polyps become numerous, making individual polyps difficult to check, the patient can be admitted for a short procedure under anaesthesia to remove them. Those who have undergone restorative proctocolectomy are seen regularly to check on pouch function (see p. 118). In addition to examination of the bottom end of the gastrointestinal tract, it is likely that the stomach and duo-denum will be examined endoscopically at regular intervals looking especially for duodenal adenomas (see p. 84).

Cancer family syndromes

In those families with the other inherited conditions (see p. 88), follow-up is rather different. Those thought to be at moderate risk may well be asked simply to attend for colonoscopy every few years, so that if any polyps do appear, they can be removed via the colonoscope. If breast, ovarian, or womb cancers have occurred in these families, it is likely that female family members will be offered appropriate screening of these organs at regular intervals also. Anyone undergoing surgery for bowel cancer in these families will be followed up using the same pattern as that employed in non-familial cancer patients, taking particular care to check for new adenomas or cancers in any remaining colon or rectum.

LOOKING AFTER STOMAS

It is difficult to imagine the horror of having a colostomy without the bags to collect the effluent, or the nursing and medical support to cope with learning the practicalities and problems of this new and often frightening feature of some patients' daily lives. Yet stomas predated appliances, and it is only in the last couple of decades that specialist stoma nurses have been around; sadly many areas still do not have this service.

The stoma care nurse

As mentioned previously, many hospitals nowadays have the services of a specialist nurse, known as a stoma care nurse. This important member of the team is particularly skilled in all the aspects of care of the stoma patient, from helping preoperatively to choose the best site for it on the abdomen, through looking after the stoma in the early postoperative period and teaching the patient how to look after it, to offering support and advice after discharge from hospital. The patient should ideally meet the stoma care nurse before operation. This will allow them to get to know each other, and to give the nurse the opportunity to explain and to illustrate exactly what a stoma is all about. In this way most of the fears can be dealt with and hopefully dispelled. The nurse will show the patient the bags likely to be used after the operation; he or she may show the patient pictures of stomas and appliances and may even introduce them to someone who already has a stoma to allay fears and clarify details. The patient is usually given a well-illustrated booklet as an *aide-mémoire*. Finally the stoma care nurse will very carefully choose the best site for the stoma and make an indelible mark on the skin to guide the surgeon at the time of the operation.

After the operation, the stoma care nurse will be in prime charge of training and caring for the patient's stoma problems, both in hospital and after discharge home. As you can see this is a very valuable and skilled member of the team. If a hospital does not have its own stoma care nurse it is usual for one or more members of the nursing staff to have this as one of his/her many responsibilities.

Appliances

There are many types and designs of modern appliance. They are best described by looking at what a stoma appliance has to do. It has to:

● **Act as a container of bowel motion.** Plainly the most important task. The bag has to be big enough to hold sufficient motion so that emptying need not be too frequent, yet small enough that it is not an undue encumbrance. Bags vary in size for different sized people and different circumstances; in general, ileostomy bags tend to be larger.

• **Remain adequately stuck to the skin.** It need hardly be said how important this is. Much work has gone into producing adhesives which are safe yet which do not harm the skin during wear or on removal. Many patients use a sheet of a gum called 'karaya'; this is a very useful substance which, when made up as a thin sheet, will form a water-tight seal to the skin, but which is removed easily even from sore skin. Bags can either be made with a sheet of karaya built into them, or the patient can attach a sheet of karaya around the stoma, with a plastic flange welded into the sheet to which can be clipped a bag with a complementary plastic ring. This arrangement allows the bag to be removed without taking off the karaya 'base plate', so that the skin does not need to undergo the trauma of stripping off the adhesive every time the bag needs to be changed.

Other bags use a thin film of adhesive on a resilient paper base attached to the bag. Again this can be used with a plastic flange arrangement, or the whole appliance can be removed each time the bag needs changing. This method of adhesion has the advantage of a much more pliable paper base plate, particularly useful on uneven skin, for instance when the stoma is unavoidably close to a scar.

• **The contents of the bag must be disposed of easily.** As mentioned above, the bag can be removed, with or without the base plate. Alternatively, if the contents are reasonably fluid (ileostomy effluent especially) a clip can be removed from the bottom of the bag so that it can be emptied, either directly into the toilet or into a plastic jug.

• **The wind may need to escape freely.** If the patient finds that wind is a problem, a small valve can be incorporated in the upper part of the bag which allows wind to escape without letting the fluid contents out. It has to be said that these valves do not always work very well; some patients find it better to use a bag without a valve and to make a few holes at the top with a pin.

• **The bag must not smell.** This is one of the fears most often mentioned by patients about to undergo a colostomy operation. In fact it is unusual for a smell to be apparent, though, even in the absence of smell, some stoma patients think there *is* one, detectable by all and sundry. If, however, odour does occur a simple solution is a small aerosol, easily carried in the handbag or pocket, which can be sprayed into the bag when first attached or each time it is emptied.

• **It should be as aesthetic as possible.** Lightweight, suitably designed bags made of opaque material and coloured or patterned appropriately, ensure that present day appliances are as unobtrusive as possible.

What's it like to have a stoma?

It would be silly to pretend that life is perfectly normal with a stoma. But much effort from nurses, doctors, appliance manufacturers and, very importantly, patients themselves, has gone into making life with a stoma as close to normal as possible. In physical terms, a stoma is no bar to sports (including swimming), carrying on with one's occupation, sexual activities, and having babies. Much more of a problem for some people are the psychological consequences associated with a change of body image, feeling 'dirty', and worries about 'people knowing'. In the early days, especially, the 'ostomist' (a term sometimes used to denote someone with a stoma) may have problems which seem insurmountable —the appliance may be difficult to apply, and it may leak or come away completely in the most embarrassing of circumstances. But with perseverence and experienced aid, these early problems diminish or disappear completely.

Bowel habit

A colostomy will usually evacuate into the bag with the same regularity as the normal bowel: in other words, the bag may well be empty for most of the time, requiring attention once or several times a day. If the bowel is more active than this, and this is especially likely in the early post-operative period, the pattern can be made more regular by simple medication aimed at making the stool firmer and less bulky.

Changing or emptying the bag

Bag changing is simplest if the base plate and the bag are separate, as described above; the old bag is simply detached and the new one clicked into place. One-piece appliances require careful removal, cleaning, and drying of the skin, and careful application of the new appliance; the same procedure is followed every few days to change the base plate of the two-piece version. This process is best done in familiar surroundings, but most people have a small bag of essential items with them at all times to allow them to do it anywhere that it may become necessary.

Disposal of the used bag is easiest at home; biodegradable bags are available today which can be flushed away in the lavatory. Other bags can be tied into a polythene bag (nappy [diaper] disposal bags are very convenient) and thrown away with the household waste.

If the appliance has an emptying attachment at the bottom (especially with an ileostomy), it is a simple matter to empty the bag into the lavatory, wherever one happens to be.

Irrigation (see Plate 7)

Irrigation is a very useful procedure for those who would prefer to pay as little attention as possible to a colostomy during the day. The principle is that the colon is washed out in the morning, so that the stoma does not act for the rest of the day; this means that the patient does not need to wear a normal appliance; rather they can either wear a very small bag to seal the stoma or they can just apply a small dressing, (even a small sticking plaster sometimes!) to protect the clothes.

Irrigation takes about 30 minutes. A pyramidal plastic nozzle is inserted into the stoma and a pint of water is run into the bowel from a bag held high to allow it to empty into the bowel by gravity. The fluid runs around the bowel and stimulates it to evacuate itself completely. Unfortunately this procedure cannot be used with an ileostomy. The stoma care nurse may well offer to show how irrigation works; if not, it is certainly worth asking.

Complications with stomas

Early postoperative problems

Complications in the immediate postoperative period are uncommon, occurring more frequently after emergency operations or in obese patients. They are usually the result of technical difficulties in making the stoma. The commonest complications are necrosis (death of the end of the bowel used to make the stoma) and early retraction (separation of the bowel from the skin, and return towards the inside of the abdomen). Both are serious complications. Sometimes necrosis only involves the last centimetre or two of the bowel, in which case it can be managed by careful stoma care, watching particularly for retraction; subsequently scarring may make the opening very tight, requiring operative revision of the stoma. If more than the last few centimetres of the bowel is dead, an urgent operation is needed to refashion the stoma. Complete retraction requires urgent reoperation also, as the end of the bowel emptying into the abdominal cavity would cause peritonitis.

Later complications

Skin problems   The commonest problem after the early postoperative phase is soreness of the skin around the stoma, either because of leakage of bowel motion under the appliance, or allergy to the adhesive (though this is less common these days, with special low-allergy materials). The stoma care nurse plays a very important role here, helping the patient to identify and overcome the cause and heal the sore skin. If the cause is leakage due to one of the above problems, the surgeon may need to revise the stoma before the skin problem is overcome.

Prolapse   This is extrusion of the bowel through the stoma, producing a 'spout' of bowel of variable length; sometimes it can be 6 inches or more in length. It happens because the bowel is not sufficiently adherent to the tissues inside, so that the loose bowel is passed like a stool. Minor degrees of prolapse are fairly common and pose no great problem; more troublesome prolapse may require reoperation.

Retraction   This is due to failure of surgical technique. There is not enough 'slack' in the bowel, so that the bowel end, attached as it is to the skin, pulls the skin inwards, producing a concave deformity which makes it difficult to attach the bag satisfactorily. This is most likely to occur in obese people—the stoma may look fine when the patient is lying down, but when they stand up the abdominal wall bulges forward, tending to leave the tethered bowel behind. Expert stoma care can often overcome the difficulties posed by retraction, but if the problem is more difficult the patient will find that the bag tends to come off spontaneously. In these circumstances reoperation may be necessary.

Stenosis   The opening of a colostomy is about 2–4 cm in diameter usually. Sometimes, perhaps due to early necrosis, the opening can become scarred and narrowed, so that it may be only a few millimetres in diameter—this is called stenosis. If it does not interfere with function of the stoma it does not matter, but if there is hold up with bowel evacuation it is usually necessary to refashion the stoma.

Hernia   The point where the bowel comes through the abdominal wall produces a weak spot, where there is a tendency for the abdominal contents to push outwards. If this tendency turns into reality, a hernia is the result. This shows itself as a swelling next to, or around, the stoma, caused by loops of bowel under the skin, outside the muscle layer of the abdominal wall. Minor degrees of hernia are not uncommon, but a larger hernia can be uncomfortable and unsightly, and can make attachment of the appliance difficult, leading to leakage. In some circumstances, the abdominal wall can squeeze the herniated bowel sufficiently to obstruct it or even cut off its blood supply. These are surgical emergencies, requiring urgent operation.

Reading a section like this, in which all the problems of stomas under the sun are grouped together, it must seem as though they are nothing but trouble. In fact the great majority of patients, once they have learned the tricks and gained a little experience, find that a stoma is not the dreadful ball-and-chain they may have expected before the operation.

Stoma associations

Over the last twenty years, organizations have grown up, started and run by patients, which offer advice and mutual support to those with stomas. The Colostomy and Ileostomy Associations keep in touch with the latest developments in techniques and appliances, and disseminate information and advice to their members in the form of regular newsletters and meetings. They play a particularly valuable role in counselling those about to have an operation involving a stoma; there is nothing like meeting a person who is well adjusted to having a stoma and who is back to a normal life, to help to strip away the mystery and fear.

PAIN RELIEF

Most people regard pain as the most inevitable symptom of cancer, and that when it occurs it will be impossible to control. Neither of these observations is true. Pain certainly can be a problem for some with bowel cancer, especially in those in whom cure has not been possible, but there are many ways of dealing with it, should it occur. Pain can, of course, be one of the first symptoms in the bowel cancer patient, but this section will confine itself to those patients with incurable disease, either at the time of first diagnosis or due to later recurrence.

Pain in the patient with advanced bowel cancer may be 'visceral' (arising in the intestine) or 'somatic' (arising in the muscles, nerves, and other tissues of the body). These two types are different in character, and are treated very differently.

Visceral pain

The commonest cause of visceral pain in a bowel cancer patient is obstruction of the bowel. A recurrent tumour in the abdominal cavity may involve any part of the bowel, squeezing it and thus causing obstruction. The pain is colicky, i.e. a severe pain which comes and goes repeatedly; it may be accompanied by distension of the abdomen and vomiting (see p. 83). After investigation to confirm the cause, the treatment is usually surgical—to remove or to bypass the area of bowel obstructed. Sometimes it is necessary to make a colostomy or ileostomy to deal with obstruction due to recurrent cancer.

Somatic pain

Pain arising due to cancer involving the muscles, nerves, and bones of the pelvis or the walls of the abdomen tends to begin more insidiously and to be constant. The commonest area within the abdomen to develop recurrent disease of this sort is the pelvis. This produces pain in the buttocks, anal area, or the lower part of the front of the abdomen. It may be described by the patient in a variety of ways, such as 'burning', 'gnawing', or 'aching'. If the tumour directly involves any nerves, the pain will 'radiate' along the line of the nerve: thus, for instance, it may be felt down the back of the leg.

The first task for the doctor trying to help a patient with this sort of pain is to seek to confirm the presence of the recurrent tumour and to define the exact site. The doctor will carry out a careful examination and will arrange X-rays, perhaps including a CAT scan. If a recurrent tumour is seen on the scan, it may be possible to take a biopsy under local or general anaesthesia. Having confirmed the cause of the symptoms, if curative treatment is not possible, the first line of palliative treatment is likely to be medication taken by mouth. The type of drug used will depend on the severity of the pain. Mild pain will often be relieved by paracetamol or aspirin, while moderate pain may require something a bit stronger, such as codeine, dextropropoxyphene (Distalgesic), or buprenorphine (Temgesic). For those patients with severe pain, the opiate drugs are available—pethidine, morphine, and diamorphine. While the less strong drugs are usually only given by mouth, these opiates can, if necessary, be given by intramuscular or intravenous injection. Occasionally pain in cancer patients is not satisfactorily relieved by drugs. In these circumstances it may be possible to ease symptoms using a long-lasting local anaesthetic or chemical nerve block; in rare cases it is necessary to resort to an operation to cut the nerves transmitting the pain in order to alleviate very resistant symptoms. Radiotherapy also has an important part to play in relieving pain due to recurrent cancer, especially if it involves bones or the pelvic walls (see p. 129).

Cancer patients sometimes feel that they are being a nuisance if they complain of pain, or that to use medication too readily may decrease the effectiveness of the drugs or make them addicted. None of these common feelings is true. It is important to be open about such symptoms and to talk through any worries about them or their treatment. The anxiety and depression borne of these problems make them worse. The involvement of family, friends, and medical attendants may well help to ease pain even before any drugs are prescribed. Some people have a fear of medication, and would prefer other forms of treatment for their pain. Transcutaneous nerve stimulation (TENS), acupuncture, hypnosis, and other methods may be preferable for them. Many hospitals have a palliative care team, comprising doctors and nurses who specialize in the relief of pain; they will be fully aware of the wide range of drugs and other treatments available to help with pain and, indeed, any of the other symptoms which may befall the cancer patient.

10
Postscript

Where do we go from here? What are the prospects for more effective treatments, or, even better, are realistic preventive measures in sight?

Surgery will continue to play a central role in treatment for some years to come; during that time it is likely that the movement to minimize the magnitude of operations while maintaining the chances of cure will continue and grow. It is highly likely that adjuvant therapy to improve on the results of surgery alone will come to fruition; American doctors would have us believe that we are amidst an adjuvant revolution at present, though many British doctors take more convincing of this. Meanwhile, it is important that doctors and patients play their part in advancing our knowledge of the usefulness or otherwise of different adjuvant therapies, by joining in clinical trials which compare them scientifically.

The gene responsible for familial adenomatous polyposis has been identified and its precise function will be ascertained soon. Then we may be in a position to counteract that function in a way which may alter the development of the features of the disease. At that stage, the major question will be whether that step is of any relevance to the management of non-hereditary ('sporadic') cases of bowel cancer. Other oncogenes (cancer-causing genes), and the chemistry of their products, which play a part in the development of sporadic bowel cancer will ultimately succumb to the energetic curiosity of the molecular geneticists and biochemists. And then we really should be in a position to muzzle the disease and perhaps even prevent some cases.

While these promising scientific endeavours continue, what can we do as a society and as individuals to minimize the risks associated with bowel cancer? It may well be that screening, using the relatively crude faecal occult blood tests at first, while more efficient methods are developed, will be shown in clinical trials to decrease the population-wide rate of fatal bowel cancer, after which national screening programmes may be instituted. It is unlikely that very solid evidence of the beneficial effects of dietary manipulation will be produced in the near future, as the science of dietary study is so difficult. Many people feel, however, that eating a 'healthy' diet is at least acceptable and perhaps even enjoyable, so they will hope to decrease their personal risk in that way.

Many have written down the decades, often more in hope than in realistic expectation, that the time when we will conquer cancer is close. But it really does feel today as though our basic understanding of malignancy and its causes is reaching a point at which we will be able to alter fundamentally the course of the disease by methods less crude than surgery. Bowel cancer will almost certainly be one of the first major forms of cancer to succumb to the scientists, doctors and patients working towards that day.

Index